The Zodiac Angels
for Capricorn

Other publications by Dr Heather Parsons

The Colour of Angels

Daily Messages from the Alchemy Angels

Atlantis Revisited

The Gem Within the Soul

Dining with the Angels

Magic and Fables From a Land Time Forgot

This Shining Light

The Angels of World Peace Cards

The Zodiac Angels for Scorpio

The Zodiac Angels for Sagittarius

The Zodiac Angels for Aries

The Zodiac Angels for Pisces

The Zodiac Angels for Taurus

The Zodiac Angels for Gemini

The Zodiac Angels for Cancer

The Zodiac Angels for Leo

The Zodiac Angels for Virgo

The Zodiac Angels for Libra

The Zodiac Angels forAquarius

All available from www.angelsrus.co.uk

© Copyright Heather Parsons 2014

All rights reserved. No part of this publication may be reproduced, stored in any retrieval system, or transmitted in any form or by any means, electronic, mechanical or otherwise without the prior permission of the copyright owner.

Cover design by Heather Parsons.

Published by angelsrus, Somerset, UK
www.angelsrus.co.uk

ISBN 978-0-9931264-1-3

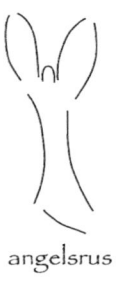

angelsrus

About Heather

Heather Parsons spent her early life in science research being awarded a PhD for her work on drugs to treat cancer. Heather then lectured in Biology in various colleges and for the Open University. Her life changed forever after a diagnosis of cancer when her daughter was only two. Her knowledge about cancer and her growing awareness of alternative medicine gave Heather the impetus to use visualisation and breathing techniques to try to remove the cancer.

After this event Heather chose to retrain in complimentary medicine and after four years she began to see and feel the spirits and angels around her especially as she worked on people. Heather began to paint these images with their swirling colours and at present has painted over a thousand images from the spirit world. Heather's scientific training has given her a unique insight into explaining the world of energies at a level where most people can understand the concepts involved.

Heather is married, lives in Somerset, has a daughter at university and a very lazy schizophrenic cat.

Contents

Letter from Lord Kuthumi

Introduction

The Capricorn Person – poem

Chapter 1 - Challenges for the Capricorn Person

Chapter 2 - Angels of the Zodiac

Chapter 3 - The Zodiac Art Images

Chapter 4 - The Secret of Life

Chapter 5 - The Colours Within the Images

Chapter 6 - Three Groups of individuals

Chapter 7 - The Capricorn Person

Chapter 8 – Responses within the Capricorn Person

Chapter 9 - Angels of the Zodiac for Capricorn 1

Chapter 10 - Angels of the Zodiac for Capricorn 2

Chapter 11 - Angels of the zodiac for Capricorn 3

Chapter 12 - The Future

Letter from Lord Kuthumi

Every person who now lives and walks on the Earth is an amazingly courageous individual. They have been brave beyond measure to have lived before, to have fallen in love and to have stood up to their aggressors in battle. Their courage extends to experiencing all manner of trauma and all manner of deaths. The human rarely gives up hope for this illuminates the nature of the human as being able to think and believe in something spectacular far beyond what can be seen. The human knows deep inside that at some point they have to sort out their old memories and to offer love and healing to those they have wronged and to be able to forgive themselves and those who have hurt them. Along this journey the body may begin to suffer as the mind does not understand the process of returning energies and through fear blocks these memories which reverberate throughout the body. You all have allowed this fear to permeate the sides of your mind and restrict your glorious vision of freedom.

Allow love and empathy to fill your being for you are all doing so amazingly well so be proud of what you have achieved. One day you will walk away and smile at the stories from long ago and the love stories which have bound you to loved ones in life after life and you may even love the same people in this life. I salute you all and I and the spirits will be around to help whenever you call on us so please ask for guidance or inspiration as your journey reaches the high peaks one day you will smile at the journey you have undertaken and the lessons you have learnt.

Introduction

Every person is a complex mixture of ancient choices and long held dreams together with the thoughts and problems from their current life, which often throw the individual off their chosen course. The soul is the sum of all the thoughts since the very beginning of time itself. This soul is truly amazing and can bring joy, happiness and inspiration to the lives of many. This soul is our base, our sanctuary and a touchstone for the path being walked. The further along this path the person walks and the more stepping stones are jumped over the easier the journey becomes and the more in touch with the soul the person becomes. Tune into your dreams from childhood days and find out who you are. Allow these angels to provide inspiration and to guide your steps for they will never let you down and will help to transform your life. Life on the earth should not be difficult unless we have allowed old memories to infiltrate the sub consciousness, life should be full of fun and laughter with friends as we follow long held dreams.

The Capricorn Person

I am the greatest of believers and the highest of the seers
Fear though grips my insides and I like to focus of the reality of the world rather than the spiritual side for I need a focus and I need to know the answers, science gives me this
It also leaves a gap in my life which feels like an empty hole
I do not know what is missing but something certainly is
Born in the depths of the winter I am slightly distant from people yet I like them and try to organise them and help whenever I am able to
I love the palest of blues which link to the icy days of my birth and these blues bring a sense of calm which I need as I tend to be rather stress as I allow problems to build up within me
I use the water wisely for it allows me to think and to dream of better days still to come, the water brings clarity in its wake and gives me the ability to think amazing thoughts
When problems arise within me then I still try to use the water to bring clear answers but these often do not come so I try to cool the body down further, this is reflected in my muscles becoming tight and my body feeling the aches from this cooling down
If my problems are severe I can even begin to freeze my thoughts down but I still find it difficult to find the answers I once found so easily
I am the trust that never dies in the heart but within me this trust has

been lost and my challenge is to find it again

I need to believe for without faith my life is meaningless

How do I find this again as I tune in so completely to the logic and explanations that I crave

I need to find a spiritual perspective in my life but this seems almost impossible as I fear the voices and words that I sense in m quiet times

1.The Challenge for the Capricorn Person

You are an amazing spirit with dreams from long ago and dreams from yesterday to achieve and promises yet to be come. You have come to Earth with challenges to sort out from past lives. These often cloud our path and make it more difficult to see the stepping stones across the ravine. Every person can choose to tap into the consciousness of the universe or to ignore the past and become enmeshed with other problems on the ground. When did people come so fearful that they allowed this fear to creep in at the edges of their consciousness and permeate their whole being and as this fear accumulates it begins to block the light from within shining out far and wide across the world.

Every person has come down to the Earth to face challenges and these are often very testing and are often problems from past lives which we cannot move on from. The challenge for the Capricorn individual is to regain an ability to trust in the universe which will never fade for they know that their journey is eternal. This tremendous faith was lost in a previous life, maybe centuries ago in difficult times. This needs to be rekindled again for without trusting the truth which is all around them, the human spirit is limited in their goals and beliefs. This incredible believe may have been lost in earlier centuries after the spirits or your family let you down badly. This person often has issues with parents to sort out and a love to be rekindled as they may have felt abandoned and very much alone.

Without belief the Capricorn person is a little distant from others and is often hard on their loved ones and can be a tough taskmaster.
Without trust they respond with continuing to think of answers even when no answers come to light and in the process can begin to cool down the body and start chronic aches and pains. This eternal trust can be regained, maybe through the angels or spirit guides or being successful in their work and in doing so the Capricorn individual will rest easy and be able to tune in more easily to who they truly are and to begin to follow their long held dreams. Through this salvation can come about as we begin to climb high above the clouds, helping others along the way.

1. The Angels of The Zodiac

The 'Angels of The Zodiac' are the angels who surrounded us at the time of our birth. The angels reflect our personality, passions and dreams. They help us along the path we have chosen. Whatever the path, it can at times be rocky and challenging. These angels are around as we try to climb over boulders, are lost in the desert or feel exposed on the mountain side. The energies or thoughts of the angels can be shown as direct angelic images or swirls of vibrant colours with abstract images. All of the images have multiple meanings and can be interpreted in many ways. At the centre of each one though is the overwhelming universal love which surrounds us all so completely. The angels help to release problems within the left side of the brain which is the thinking logical side.

These angels come from over 1000 angels and angel energy pictures created over a 5 year period. There are many messages to be found within the angels and images so look closely and feel for the correct message for you.

The Angels of Guidance
These are the angels who find it easiest to contact the humans who walk on this amazing planet. They are often the Archangels such as Gabriel with their apparently smaller wings as if they have lowered their energies to be able to pass messages across to the humans.

These are the best known of the angels but they are only one group of angels among an enormous number of such gatherings.

The Angels of The Matrix

The matrix is the sum of all connections between individuals across all time, all countries and space. This matrix is shown by the thin gossamer threads which connect people together until the threads can be gently loosened and dissolved away. The connections could be about great love affairs and our desire to help others we once loved or about an altruistic desire to change the way we think or behave.

These angels have given us messages about our freely chosen dreams and destiny from aeons ago or from only yesterday.

The Angels of The Rainbow

The Angels of the Rainbow remind us of our destiny which has always been freely chosen in past times. These angels usually have very large wings to remind us of earlier times on the Earth when all humans could contact the spiritual world very easily. The rainbow is the metaphorical brilliance of the human who choose their destiny to help others. If we can begin to follow their guidance then the proverbial pot of gold will be waiting to be found at the rainbow's end. This is not the wealth humans crave but a far greater sense of inner serenity which comes from knowing that the best has been done and that others have been helped and justice done. These angels have given us messages about our freely chosen destiny which could have been made a thousand years ago or when we were a child in this lifetime.

The Earth Angels
These angels are all surrounded by red and blue swirls of energy for terror and a desire for revenge. These emotions, even ancient ones, hold us rooted to the spot and prevent progression more than anything else on the Earth. Most of these angels have scarlet somewhere within their swirling energy fields. This scarlet is a beautiful colour yet in spiritual terms is signifies a deep hatred which is still affecting the decisions made even many lifetimes after the events took place. This hatred and a desire for revenge against someone holds the human back in so many ways as these feelings still want to be addressed and they continually circulate and prevent a new way of thinking or of being. These angels all appear with red and blue swirling energies around them. These ancient desires can dissolve away in the depth of the nights and as they do so the body breathes a sigh of relief as it can now move on and enjoy the rollercoaster ride of a new lifetime.

The Angels of the Imagination
These are the angels who know how the human responds to problems and this response varies every three to four days throughout the year. These angels give clues over how any individual responds to problems. This response is based on the season they are born into,

the social whirl of the time of their birth, the means of their previous death and any choices they have made to be challenged in this current lifetime. The power of the imagination is truly phenomenal for it can connect us to the angels and the stars but it can also be used for the worst reasons as fear settles into the core and disturbs finding out who we are and it could also lead to self destructive tendencies. Use the imagination wisely for it can change lives. All of these images have a gentle spiral within their body. This spiral can slowly begin to spin and in so doing it can begin to break long held patterns of behaviour which have beset the person since childhood days or even from earlier lifetimes.

The Rescue Angels
The Rescue Angels are present to help protect people against rage from long long ago. There are two pillars in the body which run through the trunk and up to the two hemispheres of the brain. Rage within the right pillar is our own rage returning to the person who created the rage in the past. Rage within the left pillar is the guilt we feel over how we have affected others as we sense their rage still around especially when we meet another in this life who we think we have offended long ago.

The Alchemy Angels
The Alchemy Angels give messages and help transform our thoughts into nuggets of gold. Every angel has arrived with a positive

affirmation to help alter our destructive thought patterns and to replace them with more positive ones which can gradually become a new reality. These affirmations should be said out loud and made personal with the person's name attached to the message for this gives them greater power.

The Angels of Enlightenment
These are the angels who help people see events in a different perspective and in so doing the individual can begin to forgive others and themselves for the hurts they caused. Every person was already forgiven long ago before the mountain ranges rose high or the seas ebbed and flowed across the planet. If any person chooses to hold onto their guilt then the choice is theirs alone but this choice can prevent them moving forward into a new way of being and thinking. These angels have very serrated wings as if these serrations can begin to cut into the dark areas of our collective guilt we have long hidden away.

The Angels of World Peace
The World Peace Angels help to heal major events in the world. They can be called on to help whenever a major incident occurs. They include angels to help rescue souls lost at sea or in mining disasters or who die from famine or a tsunami or an earthquake. Whenever a major disaster looms call on the Angels of World Peace for they can help the souls of the dead to move on and can help to

rescue any still alive for they will never give up whilst any human needs help.

The Angels of Innocence

These Angels of Innocence show a fun side to life as inside us all there is still a child and a desire to laugh and be happy. They can help us to reconnect to this joyous lighter side of who we are for through laughter amazing transformations can take place as the laughter helps everyone to release their suppressing mechanisms. These are also the angels for the truly innocent person who wants to help others and often does so by naively offering them sanctuary within their energy field hoping to heal them with their overwhelming love.as the years go on though this task appears to be impossible.

The Angels of Transformation

These angels are for the person who feels they are a victim either literally or metaphorically speaking. Maybe they were bullied at school or by a boss in industry. Maybe their parents pushed them into a job they do not enjoy or maybe finances dictated the choice of a career. This is a mind set of being a victim and we do not need to carry this state forever. The angels will help us to alter the perceptions of this state and change it into a learning experience from which we can reach out to help others.

The Angels for Challenges
These angels appear with oddly shaped wings and seem to be doing wacky things and enjoying life to the full. They work particularly with the return of ancient memories which still have the power to shock as they return to the fold for there is nowhere old memories from centuries ago want to be other than with the person who formed the thought in the first place. The wings of these angels can truly delve into the darkest of our hiding places and disturb the old memories we want to hide away. With the memories in place the body will feel the aches and pains from deep within. If we allow these old memories to flow away and even to be joined back into the energy body of who we are then the body breathes a sigh of relief and yearns to enjoy the years left on the ground to the full. Not only do these angels help release old memories but they can also help to loosen physical problems which have grown within the body and are causing problems such as fibrous tissue, benign tumours, cysts or even some cancers.

The Angels of the Shifting Sands
These angels also have peculiar wings as if they are carrying a heavy burden and have been doing so for many lifetimes. These angels allow a brilliance to enter our lives as they begin to shift the sands from under our feet and bring radical changes to life. These angels can help to increase the power of the immune system to fight all infections within us and also to destroy early cancer cells which have

altered markers on their cell membranes. As they work they help to break long standing patterns which people are familiar with but which serve no one well. With these changes come a sense of relief as we now see the world in a different light.

2. The Zodiac Art Images

These images help us to reconnect with the memories that have been long suppressed and hidden far away in the core of who we are. Some of these memories form the greatest dreams we have ever had and form the basis of our freely chosen destiny. Some of these old memories may be ones which we have not liked and so have pretended they did not ever exist as we have hidden the memory far away out of sight we hope forever. These abstract images which are more confusing are present to help release problems within the right side of the brain. This is the intuitive, instinctive side and helps to connect us to the stars far above.

The Harmony Images
Inside every person walking the ground are fears from this lifetime and terrors from more troubled times. These images help us to reconnect with these ancient traumas still permeating the body, which we try to suppress and hide away for they disturb our consciousness. These images are about getting on with others and

memories which disturb many people. With these images and angels around it is possible to release these old traumas very easily.

The Art Images
These images relate to ancient fears within the energy body which the person has hidden deeply away. Whenever we can let our fears disappear then the imagination can soar to new heights and the person can be truly inspired.

The Ancestral Healing Images
Within every person on the planet are a myriad of memories from the past. Even if the person has not lived before they are still affected by the memories from their parents, grandparents and ancestors from ancient times. These old memories pass across into the developing baby just as the genes do. These old memories may show up as problems with food intolerances or allergies to foods. These ancient memories are carrying out to be heard and by being aware of these problems it is a starting point in releasing so many other problems from the lives of our ancestors and our own earlier lives.

The Images of Enchantment
These images are about loving self after so many lifetimes through hard times when words may have been said or deeds done of which we were not proud and so we try to hide these memories deep in the soul we hope to be lost forever. The energies are changing all

around the world today and it is far harder to hide memories away and so they slowly creep into the consciousness and disturb the balance of our sanity or the health of the body. Be proud of what you have already done and will continue do in the future.

The Images of Heavenly Light

These images allow us to remember old memories where all hope was lost and all dreams dashed. These images help us to reintegrate these old broken memories back into the magnificent energy body we all possess and to restore these broken energies to fullness and light.

The Moonlight Dream Images

These images relate to the person in the past who lost all hope. These cards help to wake up the blocks from numbed shock which lie around the meninges of the spine and form great barriers to the flows of energies. These images can help these old memories to dissolve away into the coolness of the breeze and bring a renewed hope back into life.

Images of Excitement

These images show how shock affects the physical body for any shock temporarily stops the flows of energies upwards. As the flows stop then the memory can become numbed and lost from the energy body and if not reintegrated will be left behind after death. In future lives these deadened memories want to be reunited with the soul who created the thought and the shock long ago. These images do not have names but numbers and within every category the colours relate to the responses of the person involved. The excitement relates to the overwhelming joy as the old memory is reintegrated back into the whole again and the energy body expands once more. Eventually when all the old memories are collected the energy body will be as it was at the start of time itself.

4. The Secret of Life

As people journey through countless lives they may lose some of the memories they do not like. These may be left behind on the surface of the planet as these troubled memories are unable to move with the positive energies within the soul into the heavens. In future lives the most difficult challenge the human has to face is to reclaim these old memories and to alter them to loving integrated ones which sit happily within the energy field of the human once more. All thoughts no matter what they are eventually want to return to the person who created the thought in the first place. If these old thoughts still have the power to shock they can be pushed away from the body and hidden in the dark recesses once more but this has an effect on their health and shows as chronic ill health problems begin to rise to the fore.

If someone died under duress then the memories within them will Flow back in a following lifetime. It is as if the person wants to be challenged to be able to accept these old memories and to forgive a demon. These old memories could relate to incredible grief, absolute rage, anger to self, guilt over a deed done or for having betrayed a friend or been a bully. These memories could also be of confusion as during a battle with gunfire heard all around or as in a asylum or a great hurt from being abandoned by a mother or left at the alter or bullied so much that the person took their own life. It is possible that a person died from poison gas and had completely lost hope of survival. Within every person walking the planet there are a myriad of memories from long ago reverberating in the energy body and making the current life appear more difficult. These past memories are like the pages of our universal story books but can only give us tantalising glimpses into our varied pasts.

The individual is always free to respond to any situation in any way they choose but some responses can have long term effects within the fabric of the body or the mind. The angel energy images help to harmonise and balance all fears and memories we have hidden deeply away. With the angels in life there is always peace, hope and the possibility of a miracle. The Angel Images help to rebalance the logical left side of the brain whilst the angel art cards help to rebalance the intuitive right side of the brain. These angels and art cards help to set us free to live life to the full and expand our horizons. Every day, in their presence, can be lived as a day of joy and pleasure as we choose to tune into who we are and are at long last able to follow our greatest dreams.

Whatever energies the human brings down to Earth with them they are present for a particular challenge which the individual has chosen to face. During life though these old energies from the past can be lost only to be replaced with fresh problems from the life they are now living giving new challenges for the lives that are yet to come.
For the Scorpio person all the angels within this book are important. Their most relevant angels and art images though come from within their own group for these are the ones that can bring about change either physically or emotionally as fresh challenges come into view.

5. The Colours Within the Images

The colours within the angel and art images are important for they give clues to long held problems. Black suggests old shocks, death, murder or suicide as numbed or deadened memories from the past return to the body. Greys give clues to depression. Browns give clues over a great struggle which is still going on. Scarlets are the colours of extreme grounding and the memories which still have the power to hold us to the spot and prevent change. Oranges are associated with passions, not necessarily sexual ones and excitement. Yellows are for joy, fun and a great inner wisdom. Dark greens suggest great stubbornness in the person. Greens are about an inner peace and serenity. Lime greens are about being in absolute harmony with strangers. Pinks are about love within the family whilst dark pinks suggest having the ability to empower others. Pale blues are about being able to trust in the inner self and of the truth whilst the dark blues suggest phenomenal courage to face one's demons and to look them in the eye. Violet is the colour of being able to see, hear or sense the presence of spirits around the person. Purples are about being afraid and also wanting revenge (red and blue together). White is about purity and stillness. Gold shows a great faith in something very spiritual. Bright indigo is about being protected and a browny plum colour is about suppressing the great dreams within the soul and turning aside from destiny. Most colours have both positive and negative meanings as shown within the table.

Within the images of the angels and the more abstract art images there are many messages to be found. These can be felt whilst looking at the swirling energies around the image or the inclusion of more recognisable features. The images mean different things to people so if your interpretation is different from others trust your own instinct and believe the messages within. There may also be messages that are yet to be found within the images. If anyone wished to use the power of choice over which images are particularly important for them then it is possible to cut out numbers from 1 to 26 and place these in a bag and let the universe help you to choose the most appropriate ones for ourselves

Colour of Emotion	Positive emotions	Blocked Emotions
Greens	Peace	Anger to self
Lime greens	Harmony	Rage to others
Pinks	Love	Hurts
Pale Yellows	Joy	Grief and lonliness
Oranges	Passions and forgiveness	Suppression of passion, lack of generosity and forgiveness
Deep pinks	Empowering others	Feeling bullied
Ochres	Wisdom	Confusion
Dark yellows	Respect	Betrayal or being let down
Turquoise	Eternal hope and stamina	Loss of hope and energy
Crimsons and purples	Strength	Guilt and worries
Pale blues	Trust and faith	Unable to trust or

		to believe
Dark blues	Courage	Terror and fears.

Colours of blocked Emotions

Colour of Emotion	Blocked Emotions
Black	Shock, murder, suicide
Plums	Suppression of the self
Dark greens	Stubbornness
Grey	Depression
Brown	Struggling
Deep purple	Terror and a desire for revenge

Colours of the Most Positive Emotions

Colour of Emotion	Positive Emotion
Gold	Wonderful spiritual beliefs
White	Purity, absolute understanding and completeness
Violet	Opening of the third eye
Pale Pink	Universal love

6. Three Groups of Individuals

Across parts of the world it has been known for over two thousand years that there are three major types of individuals. These are the groupings from within Ayurvedic medicine of the Indian sub continent but are applicable to all people across the globe.

These three groups of people still exist within every zodiac sign. The middle group are the most focused ones and see their goals clearly ahead of them. They may follow this path or they could turn away from it for a variety of reasons. These are the individuals with the most vata of all the energies. They want to help others and achieve their dreams. These were the children who sat a little apart from the group as they grew up and as they listened and watched they made choices to help others. These people wanted to be the champions of the group, either to lead the men into battle or to be fast or strong or to be the greatest thinker of all and to solve problems through the power of their thoughts. These angels and images have more of the focused blues within them for courage to follow the path.

The first group within the zodiac sign is closest to the energies within the pitta people. These are the dreamers of the world as they have always been able to tune into the energies of the universe and get inspiration from the stars far overhead or from their dreams. These people are not so focused on their goals but drift as they go through life as they find interesting diversions to keep them amused. These are the most outwardly spiritual of all the people and can produce amazing works of art, pieces of music or stories to warm the heart on the coldest of winter evenings. These angels and images tend to be brighter than the other groups as the lighter spirit world is more prominent in their life.

The third group within the zodiac signs are the closest to the kapha individuals. These people are the most sociable of everyone and only want to be at the centre of the group, listening to the tales of others and offering advice to help their friends. These people also drift as they go through life but their flow is often linked to the problems of their friends and they would never think of leaving their friends behind embroiled with their problems. In listening and giving advice they offer healing as the person is able to voice their woes and can feel calmed afterwards. These angels and images tend to be darker colours indicating that problems exist between people across the world. These how the dark blues for fears and the reds for hatred and wanting revenge.

How we live our life and make decisions is always a free choice in the world, albeit often pressurised by others. This choice though is also clouded by the memories from a variety of past lives. It is always possible to release these old memories for they bear little relevance to our lives today and in so doing it becomes possible to make different decisions in life and ones which bear little resemblance to the zodiac sign in which we were born. As we release ancient problems then the body improves and becomes calmer and more serene.

7. The Sun, Moon and Rising Signs

Everyone is aware of their Zodiac sun sign but the other two signs are equally important as they give clues over the role we are walking and the challenges we have to face. The Zodiac Angels of all of these groups are equally important to us. The sun sign is the zodiac sign at the time of our birth. The sun sign gives clues over our personality and how we interact with others and how we respond to problems and how our body becomes affected by our responses.

The moon sign and rising signs can be found out from tables or over the internet. This requires the time and place of birth to be known. The moon sign is very important as it gives clues over the destiny that we alone chose long ago. This might have been to hold a family together or to do something magnificent for others. It might have been to be the leader of men and lead them into battle or just to be the best friend it is ever possible to have. We might have chosen to heal others or to be the best musician in the world or a great philosopher.

The rising sign or the ascendant is the sign on the eastern horizon at the time of birth. This sign is most easily influenced by family conditioning and early environment in childhood and is most important until the age of about 30 when increasing confidence allows the individual to make their own choices. It gives clues over a major challenge which the person has to face in life and this early challenge is usually within the boundaries of the family union. This problem might have existed for a multitude of lives and to allow progression it needs to be gently loosened and any threads still holding to other people need to be very carefully released. If this is done by suddenly cutting the threads then the other person will be affected and can pull even harder at the gossamer ties for they have not been satisfied that the person has truly made amends for an act in the past. This sign is also sometimes referred to as the mask we wear in public and is how others perceive us to be. Breaking old patterns and walking onto fresh ground is what the human has to do and is able to do so very well. The rising sign is also how we want to be seen but at some stage this picture can be broken as we move onto higher hallowed ground on our journey to the stars.

The moon sign becomes more relevant to lives as the person ages and begins to follow their chosen journey up to the stars and beyond. In childhood days the person may dream of wonderful ideas but is then usually forgotten about as the realities of life, having a career, raising a family and being involved in the community take over for decades. It is often after the family has left home and there is now time for the self that these early dreams come back into focus. Believe in them for they are the stepping stones to being able to leave the confines of the Earth or to choose to return through altruism for others. These early dreams are so vital to who we are. These are not the dreams of suddenly waking up to find oneself a princess but the dreams that inspire the heart and reach out to others with love and perfect altruism at their core.

8. The Capricorn Person

The Capricorn person is born just after the winter solstice when the days are at their shortest and the cold has driven people around the fires. Here they wait for the coming spring and the new year ahead. It is a time of reflection, of thinking of the future and of gaining the confidence to do new things in the year ahead. Capricorn symbolises old age and many lives lived to the full and a plethora of experiences to fill many novels. These people are usually introverted, responsible, serious and practical with a dry sense of humour. The Capricorn is one of the great inventors of the world through their knowledge of science and being thoroughly grounded. These souls, more than any other, have the gift of clairsentience and knowing the truths of the world and morality. Their logical left side of their brain often pushes these feelings away as they cannot be explained.

When the Capricorn loses sight of who they are emotional problems show as being stubborn and obsessed with rules. In their darkest hours depression may overwhelm them. The colours of this time of the year are the pale blues of the ice covered landscapes of the depth of winter. The Capricorn is associated with the social energies of great gatherings in the depth of the winter such as Christmas and new year. The Capricorn person metaphorically likes the coolness of the winter as this coolness clarifies their thoughts. They patiently watch the world around them and learn how to manage others for future roles as organisers of others.

Their natural energies peak around 5 – 7 am in the early morning as the Capricorn wakes with a bounce for the day ahead. If energies plummet in the early morning then there is a problem with blockages in the channel and a loss of faith within the core.

The Angel of Transformation for the Capricorn Person

Moonbeam is one of the Angels for Transformation especially for the person who feels they have lost their passion and faith in life.
This angel is surrounded by a brilliant light which can brighten the darkness for so many others. One of the problems with the Capricorn person is that they have at some stage in this lifetime or a previous one lost their faith and have nothing to believe in. This though is an illusion and not the reality of the world we live in now. It is possible

to change our reality and expectations as our minds shift and hope once more springs into view.

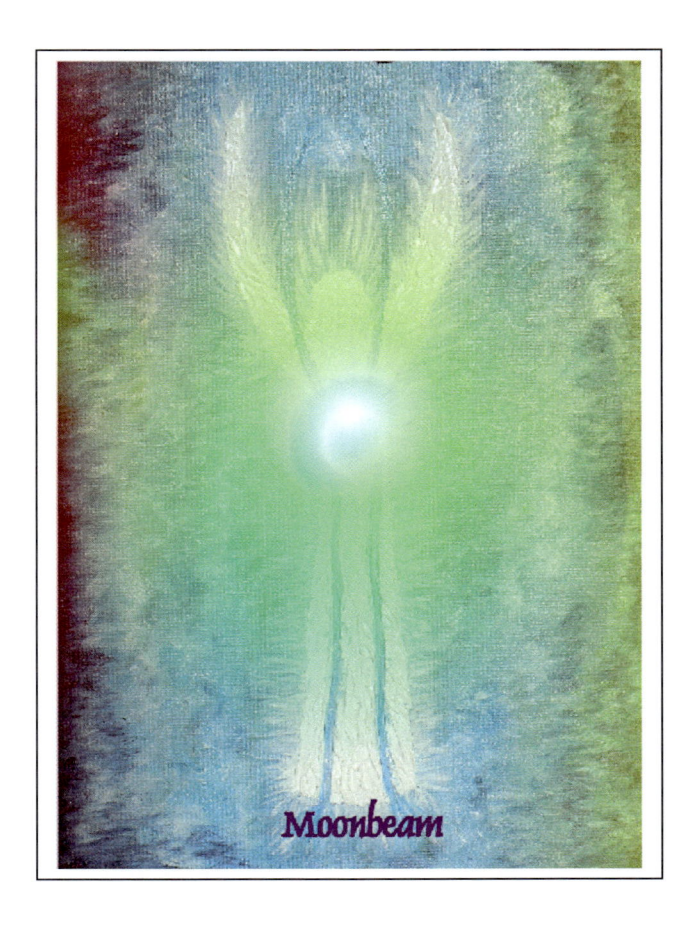

Moonbeam

There is one of the most important angels of transformation called Flame and she can present any picture to the world just as the human can. This Capricorn person has chosen to block her amazing light and power with the red crossing ribbons of energy which cross and begin to block the flows of wonderful memories and the most amazing energies upwards.

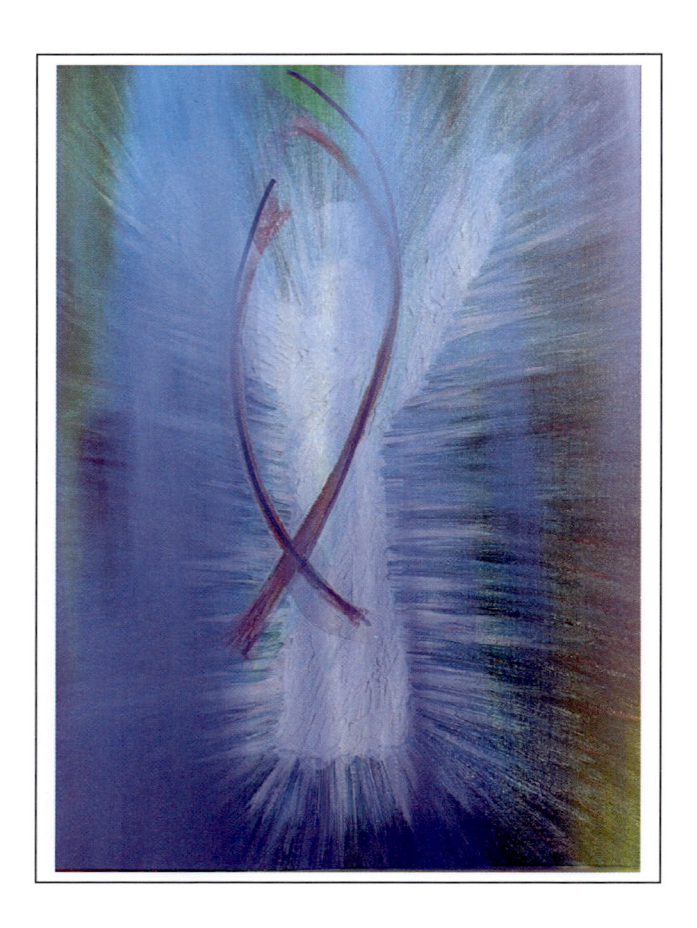

This person fears the truth that they can do amazing feats and instead chooses to walk firmly on the ground with everyone else. Within her though is the lost faith from ancient times or from last year.

As long as the person blocks their wonderful light then these lost hopes remain lost and forgotten but still has the power to leave a darkness within the soul. The blue waterfall shows how this person responds to problems as they try to cool their thoughts to find amazing clarity and the answers they crave.

Art Images for Excitement

Whenever the human experiences a major shock their energies flowing throughout their bodies become static at least temporarily. These numbed thoughts can remain stuck around the meninges of the spine for many lifetimes and cause rigidity of outlook and loss of flexibility both at an emotional and a physical level. There are a few cards of excitement for the shocks experienced by the Capricorn person. The excitement is of the wakening up of the old numbed memories and allowing them to flow and to be reintegrated once more within the energy body of the human. For as they enter the energy field the person once more begins to feel at ease and complete. As the energies flow within the human they can become reintegrated into the energy body of the whole leaving the person full of the most wonderful positive energies and able to achieve truly amazing deeds

117. This card for long term shock reminds us of a time before shocks were ever felt, a time when energies flowed smoothly throughout the body easily. The shields are present to protect the person from further hurts but in the process also lock in old injuries and trauma from long ago.

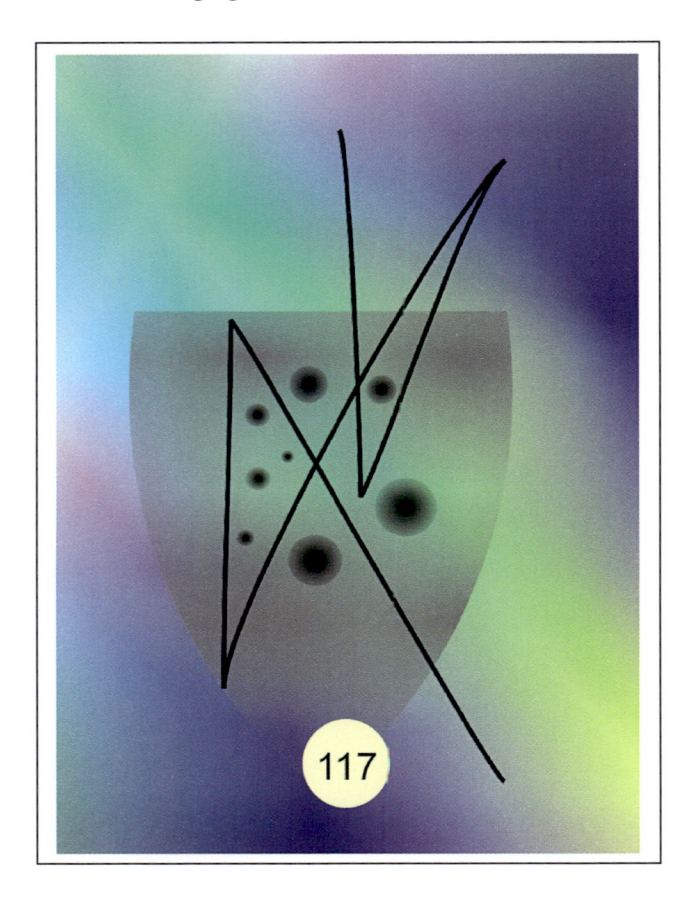

9. Responses Within the Capricorn Person

The Capricorn is inspired by the coolness and clarity of water. This is needed to hydrate their thinking brain and the water brings a sense of coolness and clarity and with this comes the answers to their problems. If problems build up then they continue to cool the water down in an effort to get the answers but the answers do not always arrive and the waters become cold or even frozen in their efforts to inspire and the body feels the effects from tight muscles to problems with the kidneys. The energy channel most important to the Capricorns is the kidney channel from Traditional Chinese Medicine. This channel is about having the confidence to do whatever is needed in life and being able to trust that this is their correct path.

Capricorn is associated with the energies of Saturn which comes with endurance, perseverance and wisdom for the ways of the world. As these people have usually blocked their right side of the brain then this imbalance throws them easily off course allowing logic and stubbornness to take hold.

This is a very important image to help bring perfect balance to the Capricorn person. Over time they have allowed confidence and trust to fade away into the descending gloom. Their clairsentience gives them a great responsibility to do something for others but this may be lost. There is always trust to be found and still time for love to flow for as the sharp spikes soften the incredible inner love can now begin to reach others as lives can be miraculously changed

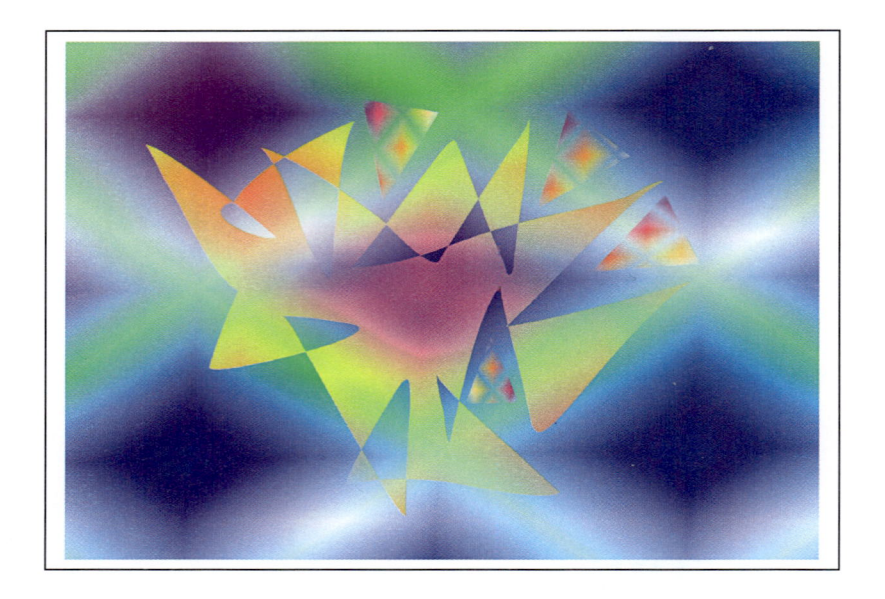

10.The Zodiac Angels for Capricorn 1

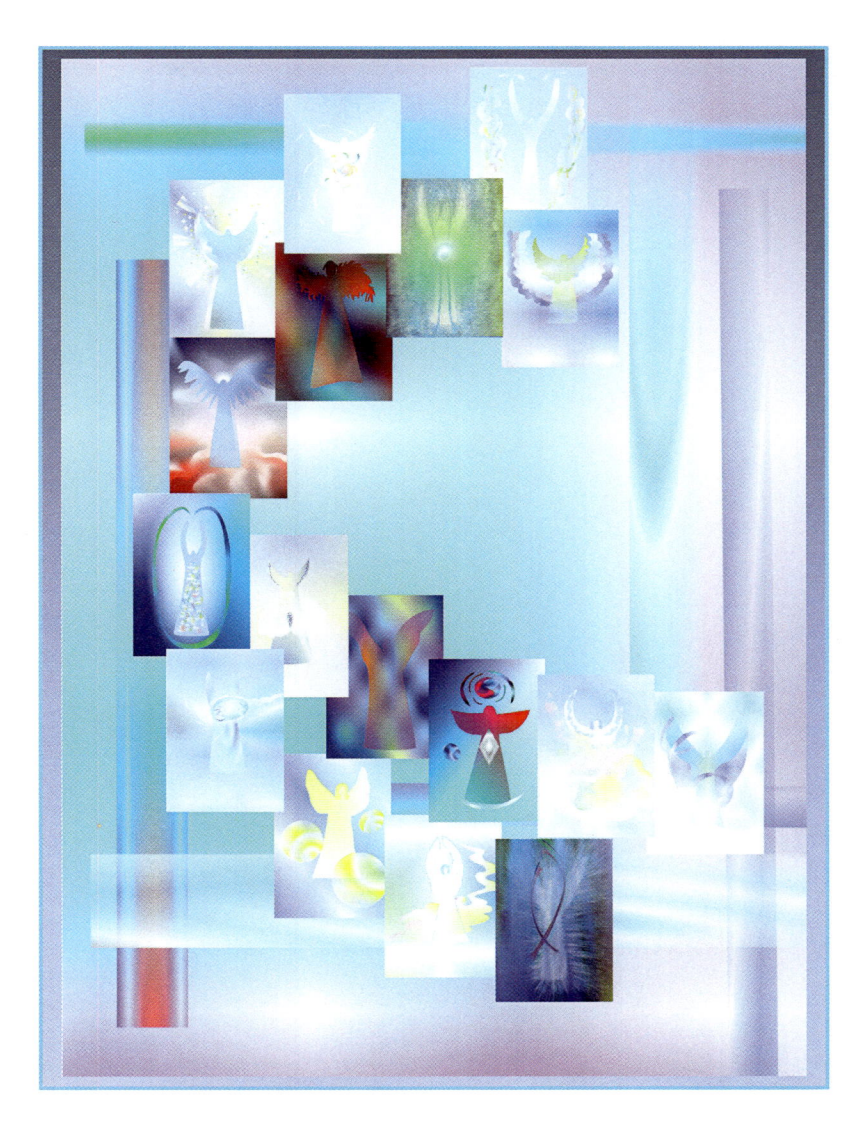

The Zodiac Angels for Capricorn 1

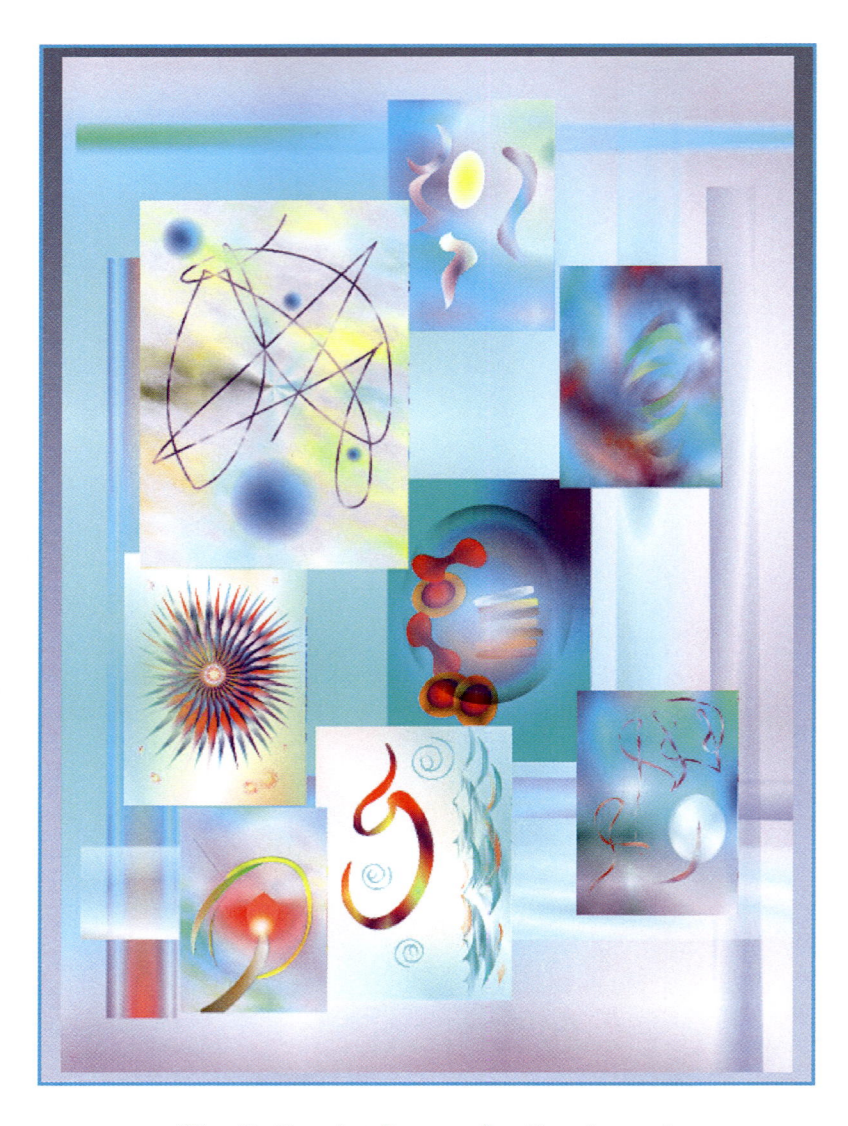

The Zodiac Art Images for Capricorn 1

The Zodiac Angels for Capricorn 1

The Energy of Mimulus

The energies of this time of the year are similar to the energies of the mimulus. The mimulus plant is a perennial growing in moist or even wet soils. The flowers are commonly called the yellow monkey flower and have a bilateral shape with a larger lower lip. These plants have the ability to grow in toxic areas such as around mine waste where other plants cannot grow. They can also concentrate salt and the plant has been used by native Americans to flavour food. This plant, like the Capricorn individual, can deal with the poisonous conditions around them and render them safe. These energies are about facing the truth and going forward with confidence.

'I face my demons with a quiet courage and a sense of humour'

The people born at the beginning of Capricorn are the most spiritual of the Capricorns and easily know the ways of the world and instinctively know how to behave.

1. Allyance is one of the Angels of Guidance. Allyance helps people to bounce back after shock or trauma. She can give support for a physical injury and helps to loosen the shock within the psyche. Her presence is always around after trauma and can offer brief moments of respite in a turbulent world. Her spinning golden energies reach out to help heal the wounds within the body.

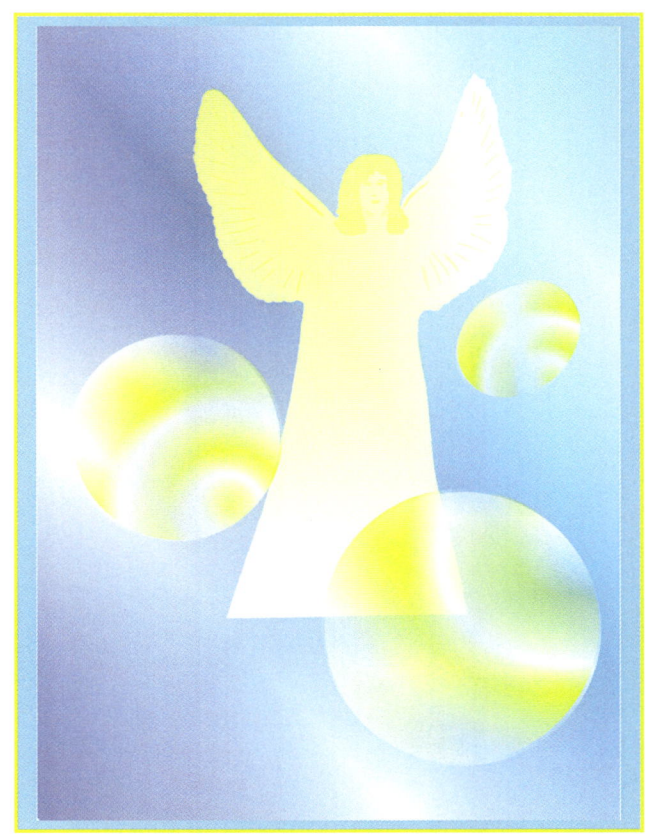

Allyance the Angel of Recovery

Allyance helps people to bounce back

after shock or trauma.

She can help to reduce the problems from a

physical injury and helps to loosen the

shock within the body.

Her energies reach out to heal

old wounds within the body

She reminds people of the joy and

the perfection of the soul which

although frail in this life is vitally

important to us all.

2. **Amazantine** is one of the Angels of Guidance He is the angel of decisions. Amazantine's presence is around whenever a difficult decision appears in life. He helps to clarify the path ahead and gives the surety of knowing that the path, although it may be difficult, is the right and only one to follow.

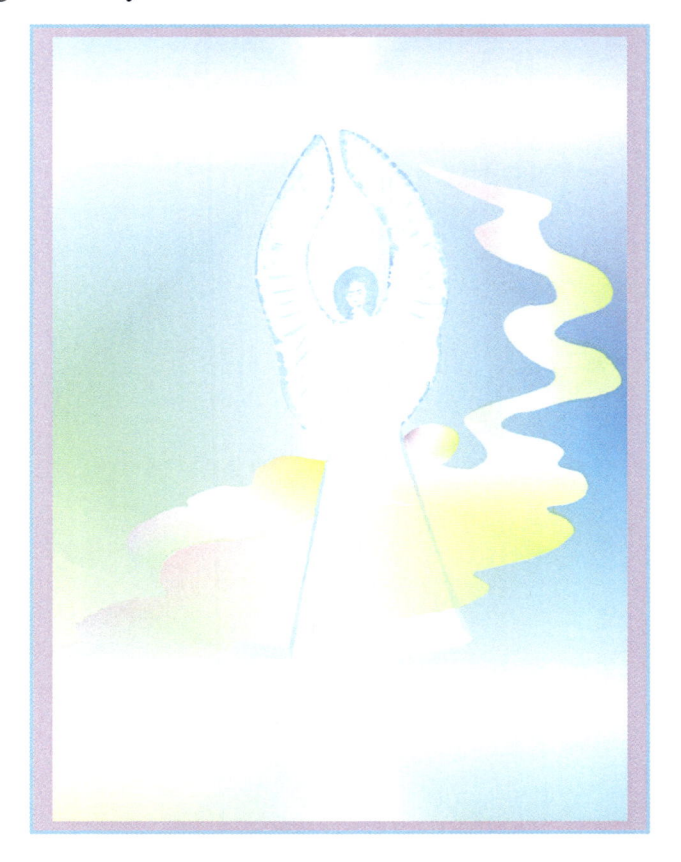

Amazantine the Angel of Decisions

Amazantine appears whenever a difficult

decision has to be made.

In particular he appears for the person who knows

they have no real choice as they have

to help or support others.

Amazantine helps clarify the path ahead

and the further this path is walked the

easier the road becomes.

3. Ariadne

Ariadne is one of the powerful Angels of World Peace. Ariadne is the rescue angel who more than others help heal personal shocks. This could be a shock of seeing an accident or hearing of the death of a close friend. In all of us shock temporarily paralysis our thoughts and actions. Ariande is the rescue angel for emotional shock. She helps to calm the mind and brings life back to the areas numbed at the news. She helps us to remember the love and joy our friends gave us and to know that they touched our hearts in wonderful ways.

The energies of Ariadne are similar to those in homeopathic 'arnica'. This restores calm after a shock either a physical one with bad bruising or an emotional one which numbs to the core of our being.

Her message is

'love yourself and your body for it houses a glorious soul'

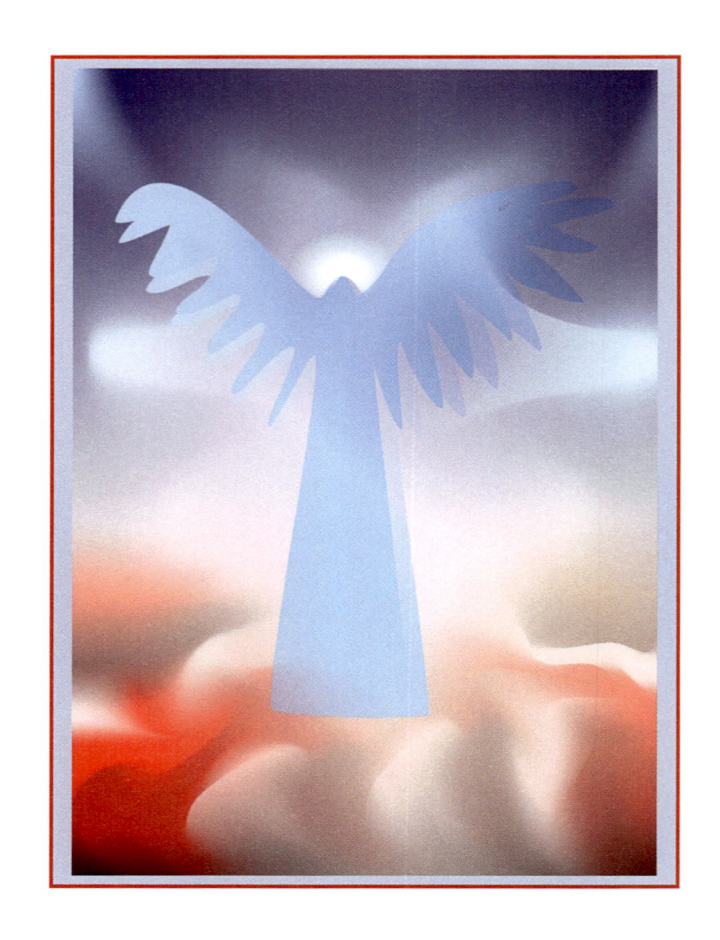

Ariadne

4. Chrisiline is one of the Angels of the Matrix and of the early days on the planet. She is the angel of optimism .tall pale blue, like blue lace agate. She is present to help the injured baby or child who still feels the need for protection and love.

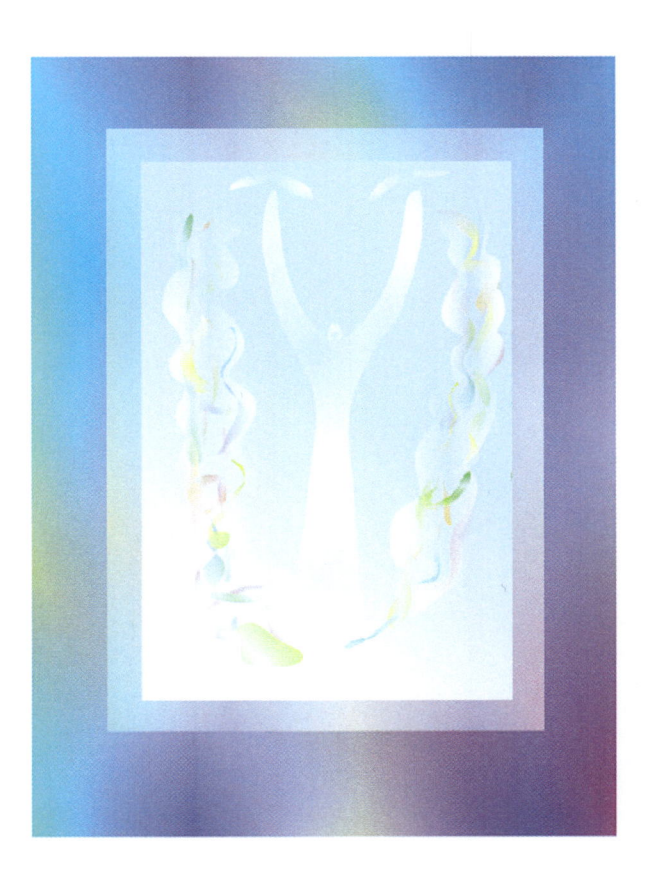

5. Clorfie is one of the Angels of the Shifting Sands who can help us to turn life around if we so desire. Clorfie helps to remove terror from the immune system so allowing us to be healthier.

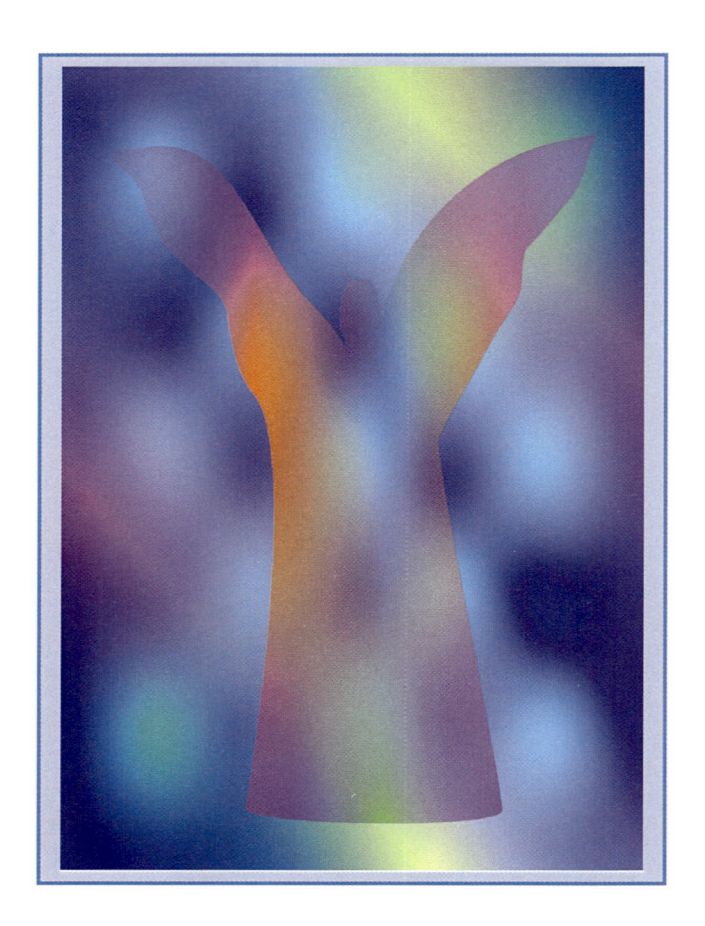

6. Codelia is one of the Alchemy Angels who have the power to transform our thoughts into nuggets of gold.

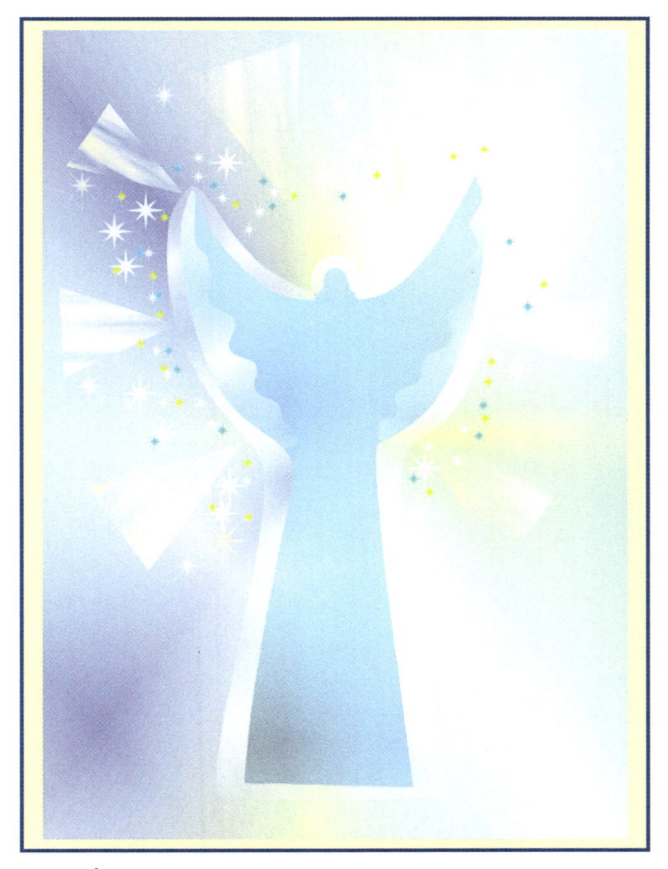

Her message is

'remember the universe loves you even when times are difficult'

7. Curiosity is an image of enchantment for the soul who feels curious about the world. This person though is a logical left brained individual who tends to ignore the intuitive right side of their brain.

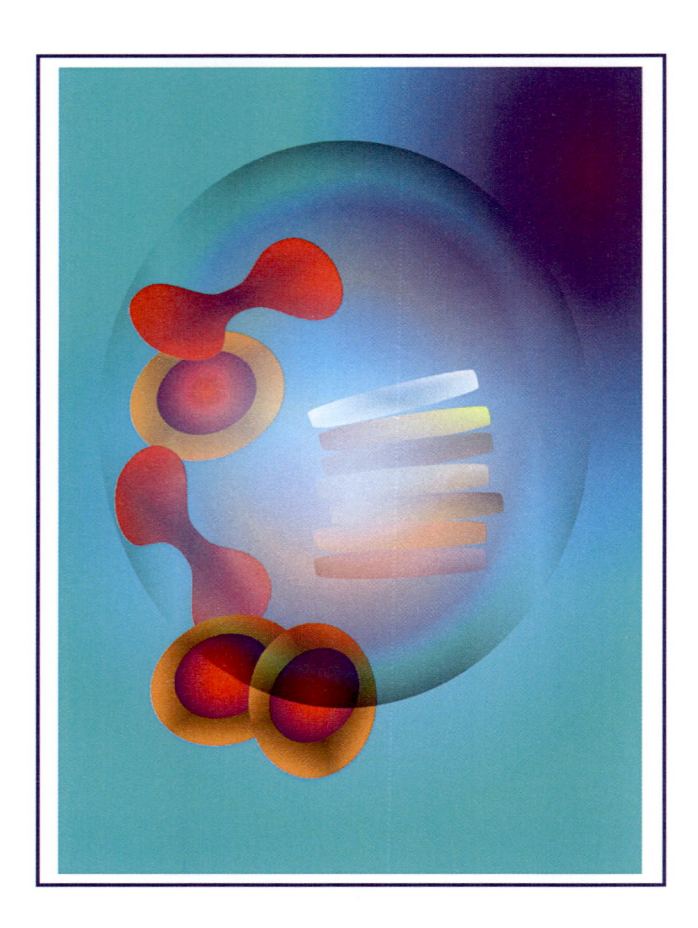

8. Direction is an art image for the soul who feels alone gazing at others within the shoal who stay together for safety in numbers. This is a brave soul prepared to stand up to be counted.

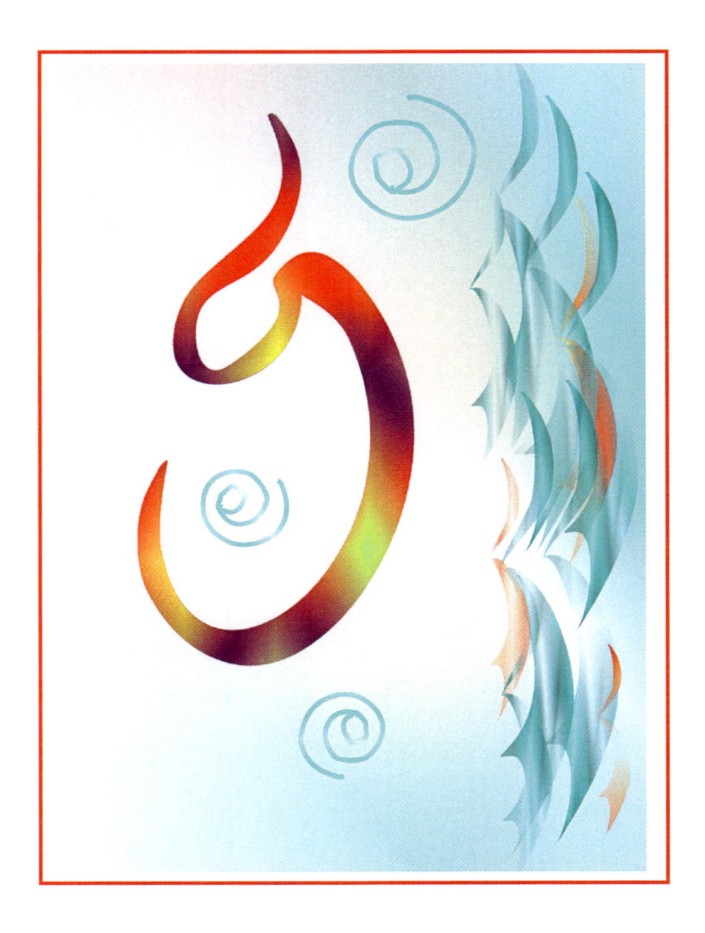

The direction is often difficult to find for these people as they know a great deal and often swim against the tide as they do their own thing.

9.Dreams is an art image for the soul who tries to ignore their dreams. Be true to these for they are valuable glimpses into another world and are a part of your bedrock and salvation.

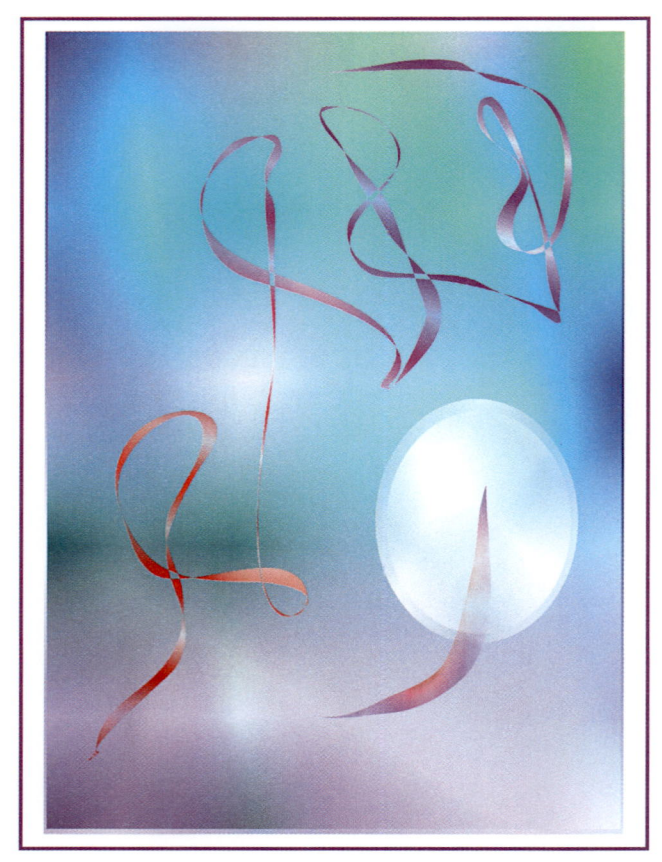

Within dreams can come images of a past life, of success and glory, of meeting again loved ones who have died or tremendously exciting dreams such as swimming with dolphins. These dreams are often magnificent and can lift the life from the humdrum to the spectacular.

10. Forellia is a heavenly light image for the soul who has lost hope of ever being able to face their innermost demons and so continues to push them away. Remember the greatest fear is fear itself and any nightmares during sleep can led the person down an important path.

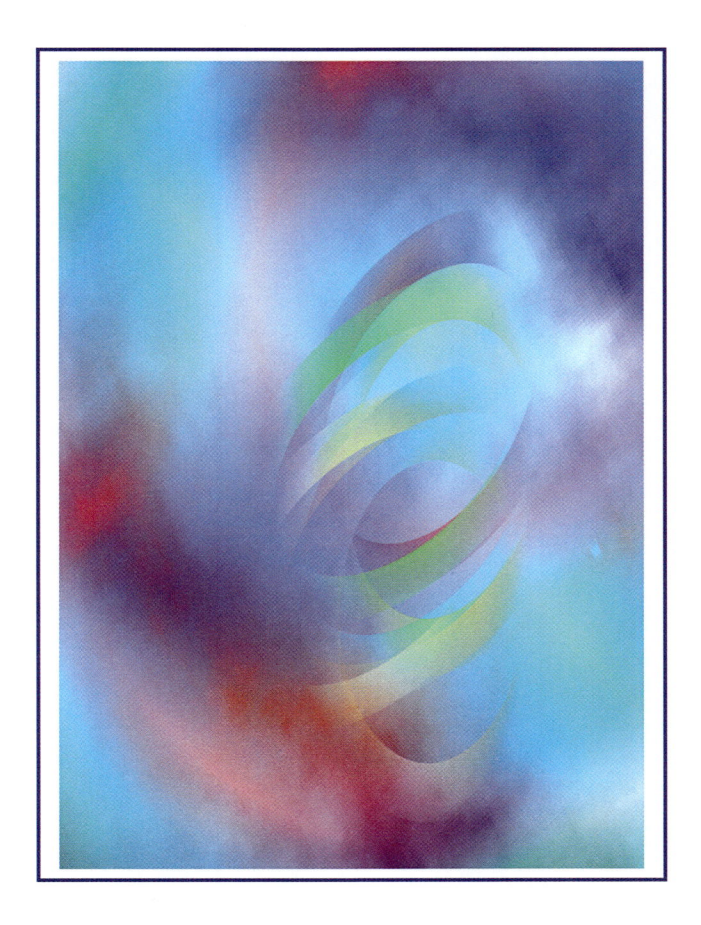

11. Fusion is an enchantment image for the soul who has great gifts but their early experiences have shattered their core. This is reflected by their spiky nature which tends to push others away.

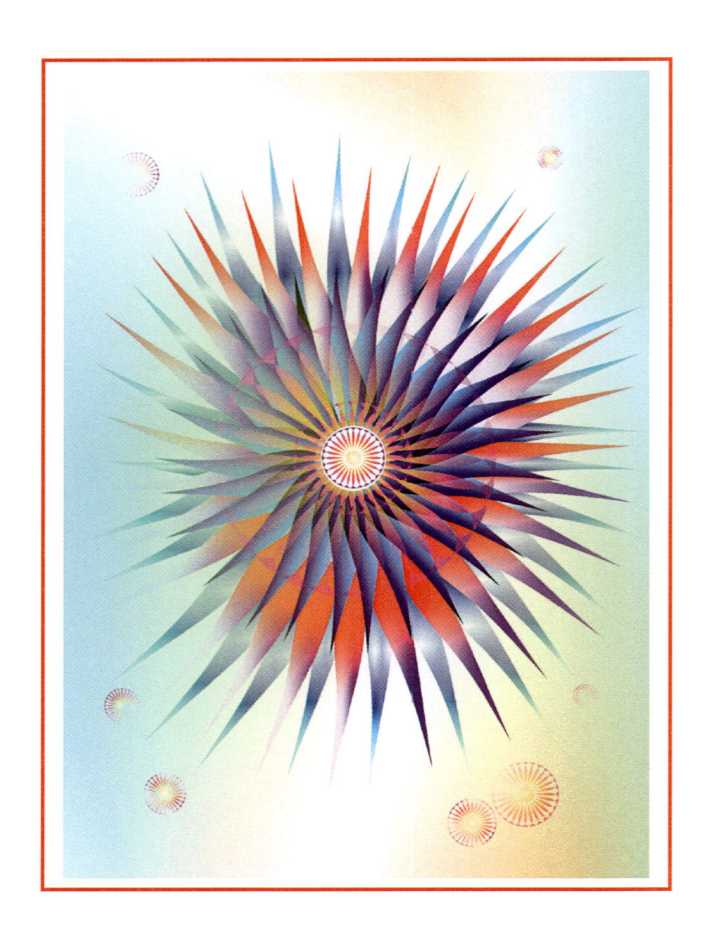

12. Happiness is an art image for the person who feels this state of being eludes them. These are the thoughts of light, joy, dancing in the spring breeze and watching the feathers or ribbons float on currants of air. Happiness is the inner child within us all.

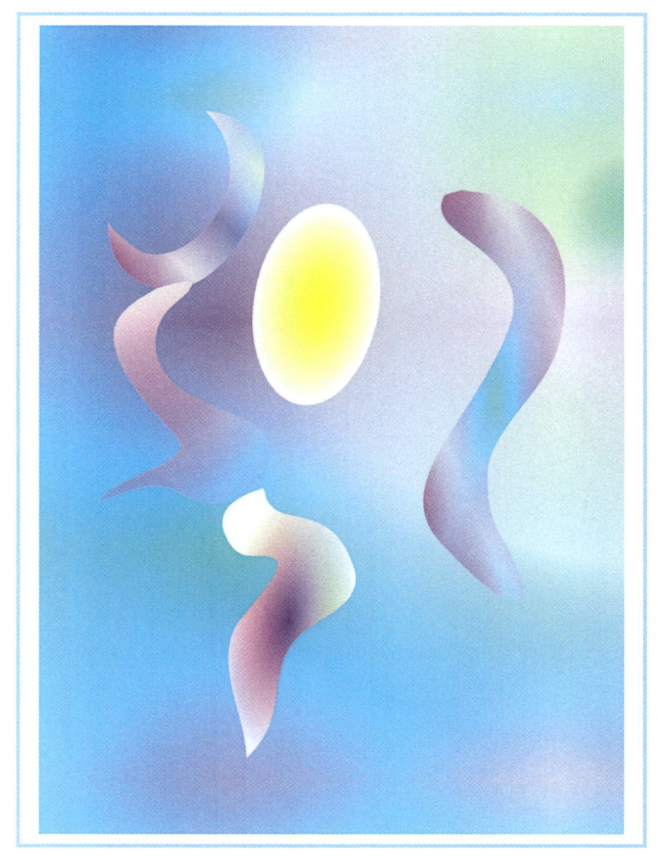

It is the total self obsession with examining a flower or watching the raindrops run down the glass or jumping into piles of fallen autumnal leaves.

13. Jolitee is the Angel of the Imagination for the soul born between Dec 25th and Dec 28th. This angel has a core of terror which takes energy to hold the core in place and if you listen carefully there can still be answers on the breeze and thoughts which settle in the mind.

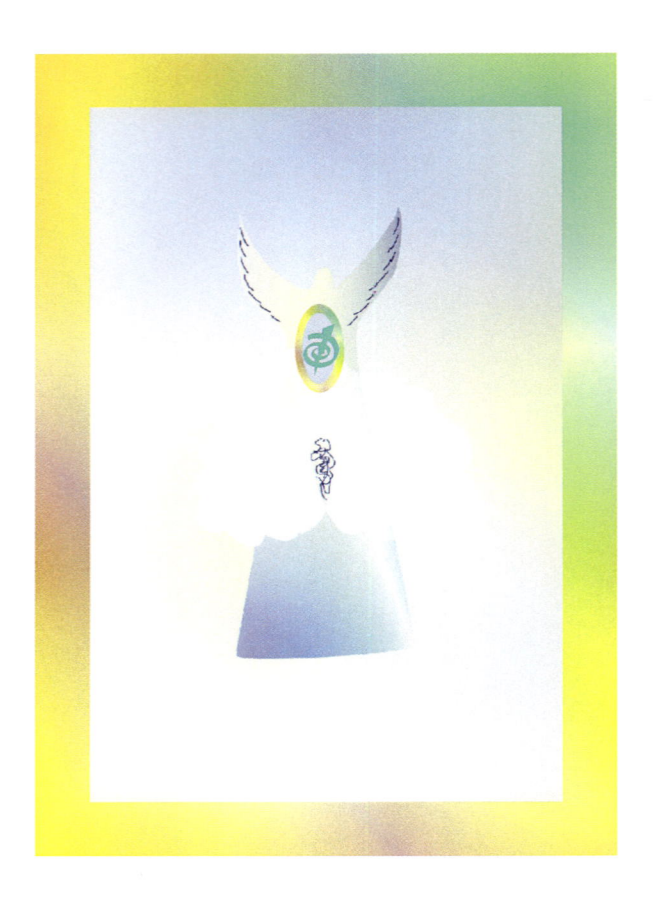

14. Khamel is one of the Angels of the Matrix and of the early days on the planet. He is for the brave at heart, the soul who has the clairsentience of the Capricorn but also the practicalities of the grounded soul. They have massive energies and abilities to help others sweep away the debris around their lives. Do not fear this role for you are well able to

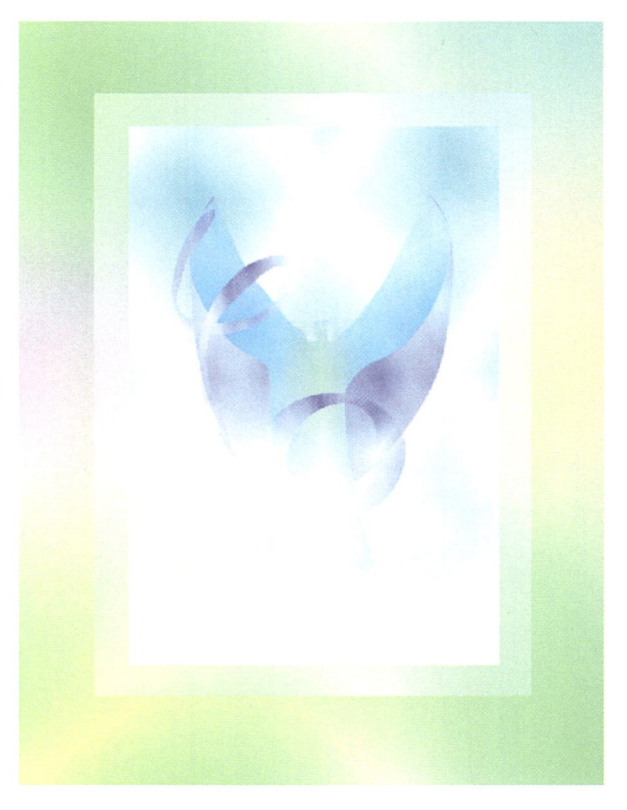

15. Kindness is an ancestral image for the soul who wishes to bring a stranger into the fold but fears the consequences. The soul may wish to give to the beggar on the street but logic tells them the money will be spent on alcohol and so this soul does nothing. Not everything is as clear cut as this soul believes and sometimes a charitable gift can set both souls onto a different path.

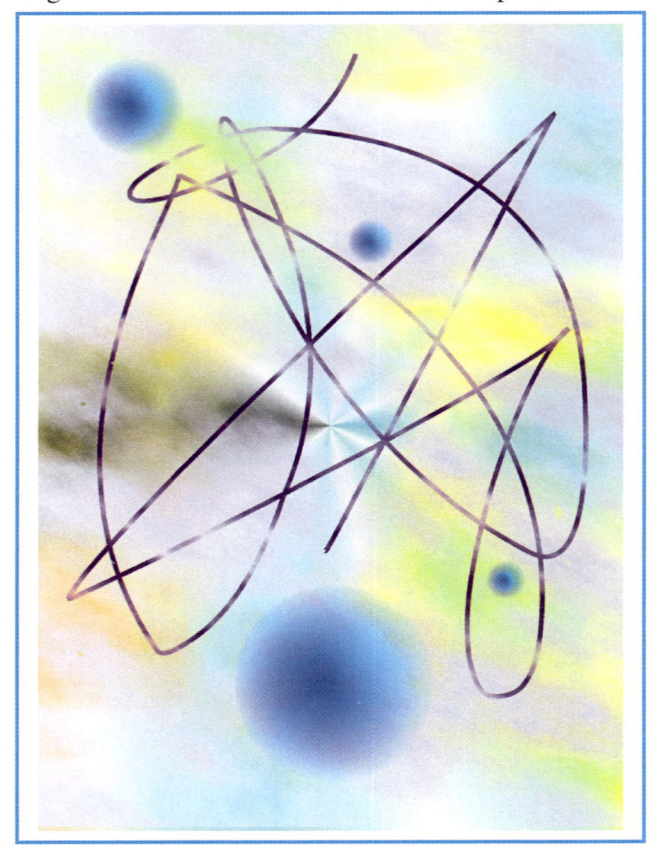

Kindness is always paid back in kind at some time in the future.

16. Lauralie is one of the Angels of the Matrix and of the early days on the planet. She is present to remind you of the greatness of your soul and of wonderful early lives. It is possible to return to this state at any time. This soul may feel that their self imposed exile is necessary but the angels feel differently.

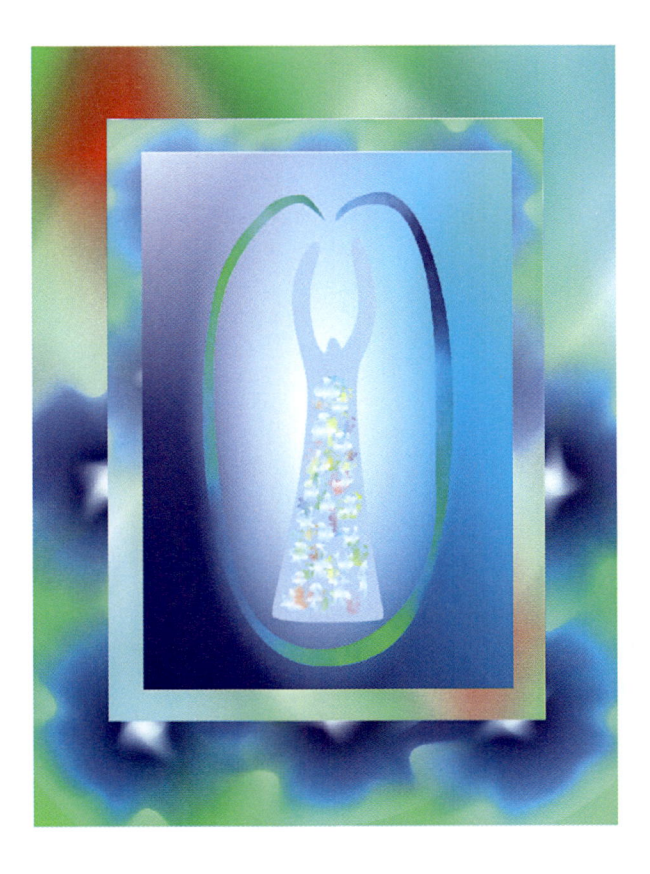

However later lives turned out they were learning experiences along the way before this soul could return to the highest.

17. Malpurnia is the Angel of the Imagination for the person born between Dec 29th and Dec 31st. The imagination of this soul tries to expand their being but others try to dampen their way. Fear restricts others and can spread to this soul as well if allowed to. Allow others to follow their own journey as you tred your path for there is plenty of help along your road.

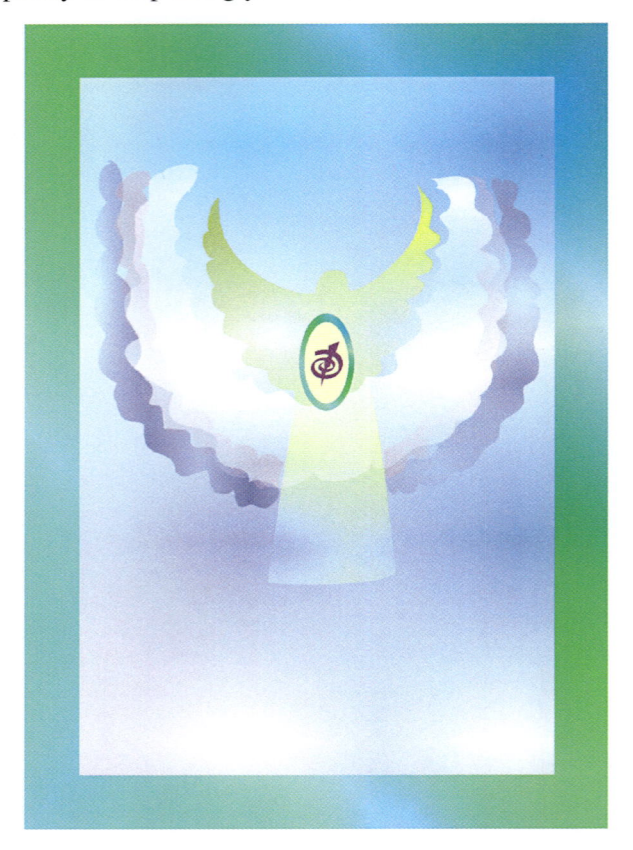

18. Marillo is one of the Angels from the end of the Rainbow where the pot of gold is to be found. This angel contains a wonderful seed which is waiting to hatch out and spread around the world.

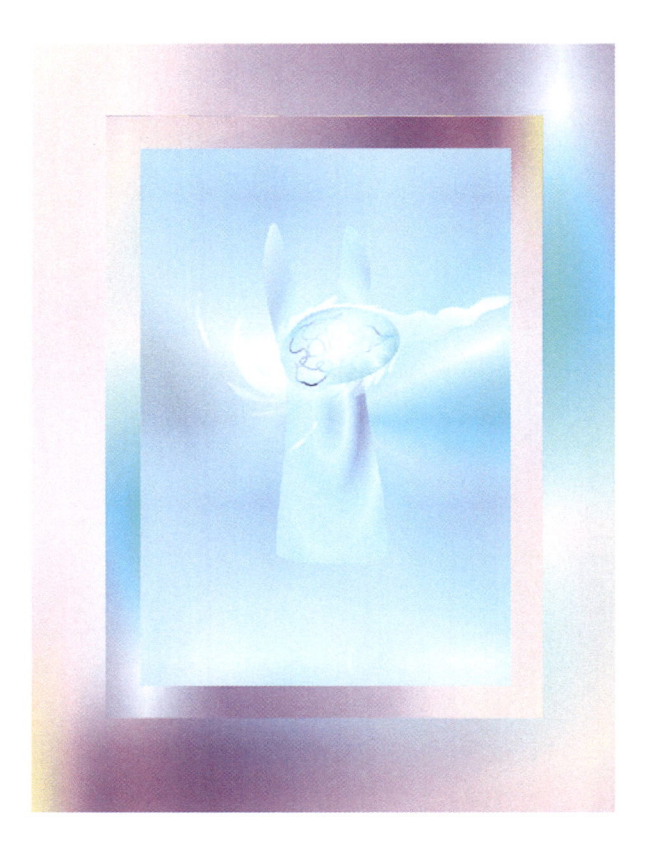

19.Mercius is one of the Angels of our Challenges which we have chosen to face in this life. The challenge here is to loosen the tightness of fears within muscles using the feather boa to low the tightness away.

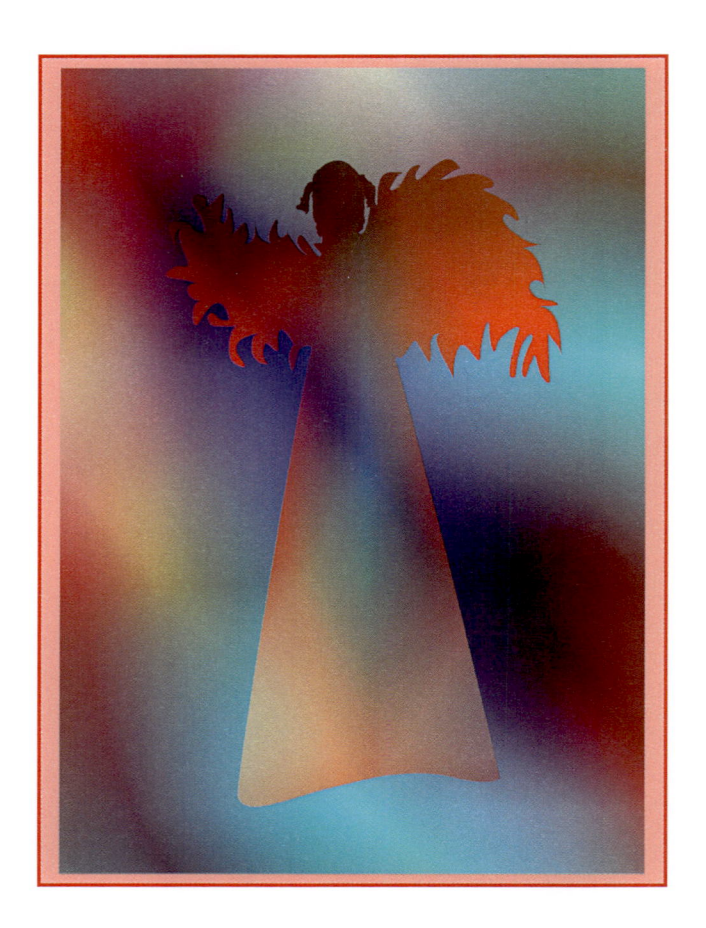

20. Merino is the Angel of the Imagination for the soul born between Dec 22nd and Dec 24th. This person still feels hurt inside due to early hurts as a baby. This soul may feel unloved because of early experiences but the truth is that they are well much loved both on the earth and from the heavens. Allow these gentle thoughts to slowly infiltrate your consciousness for they are the truth.

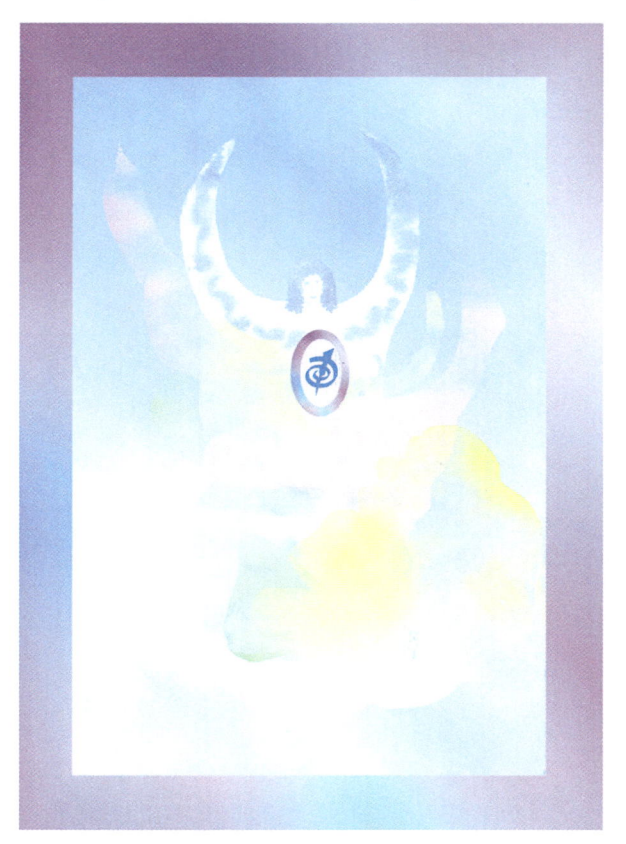

21. Pareth is one of the Angels of Innocence and of childhood days when life seemed easier and the world new and exciting. These are the angels of sharing with friends and the sheer enjoyment of the simple things in life such as conjuring up tricks to please the mind and the audience.

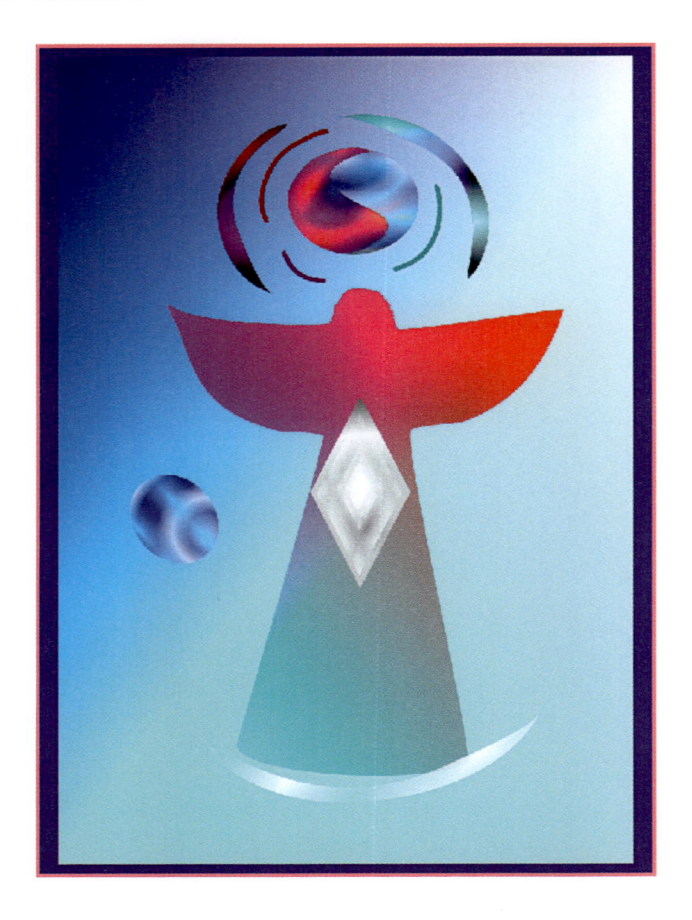

22. Sacrifice is a harmony image for the soul who has excuses a plenty for not following their path. They feel they have made enough sacrifices for others and have been unable to do what they themselves wanted. This person often feels that sacrifices are necessary to help others even if they are injured in the process.

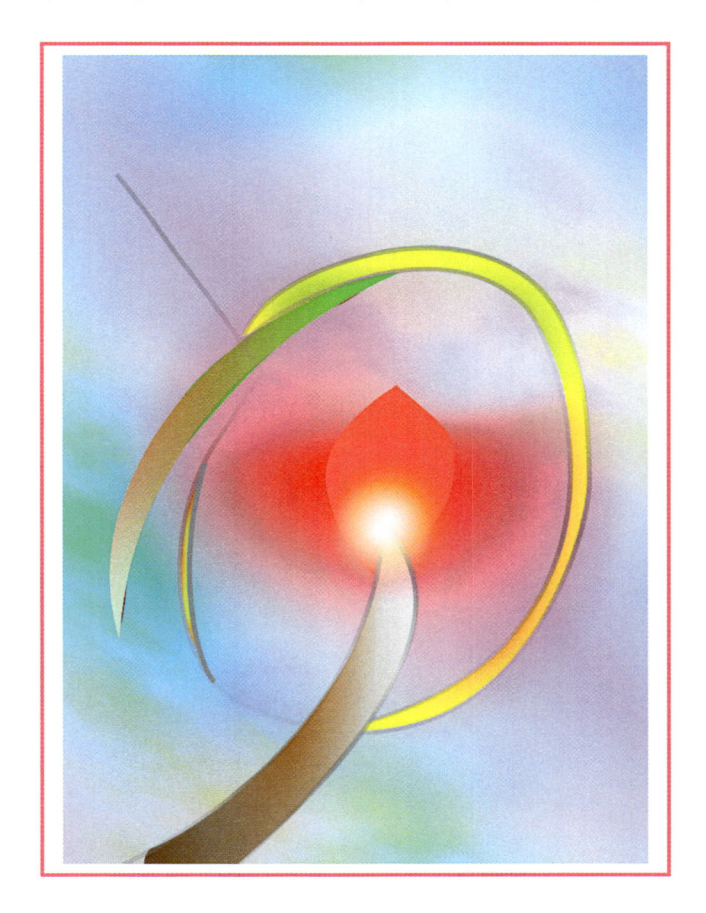

23. Swirl is one of the Angels of the Matrix and the early days on the planet. Swirl appears for the person who has chosen to follow the medical route for some illness rather than being responsible for their own ill health problem

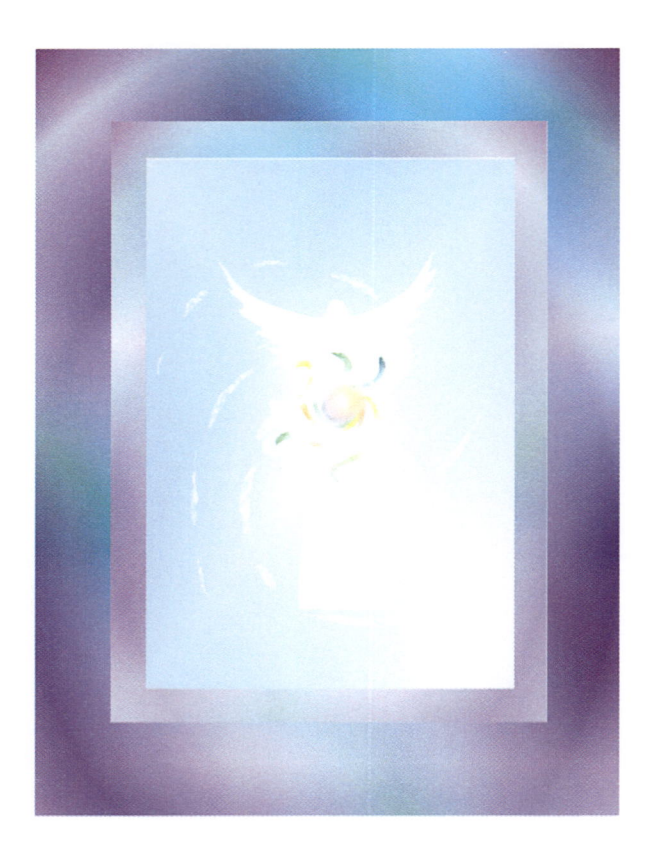

Images of Excitement

3. This image shows the tight sutures of the skull or pelvis which are unbalanced.

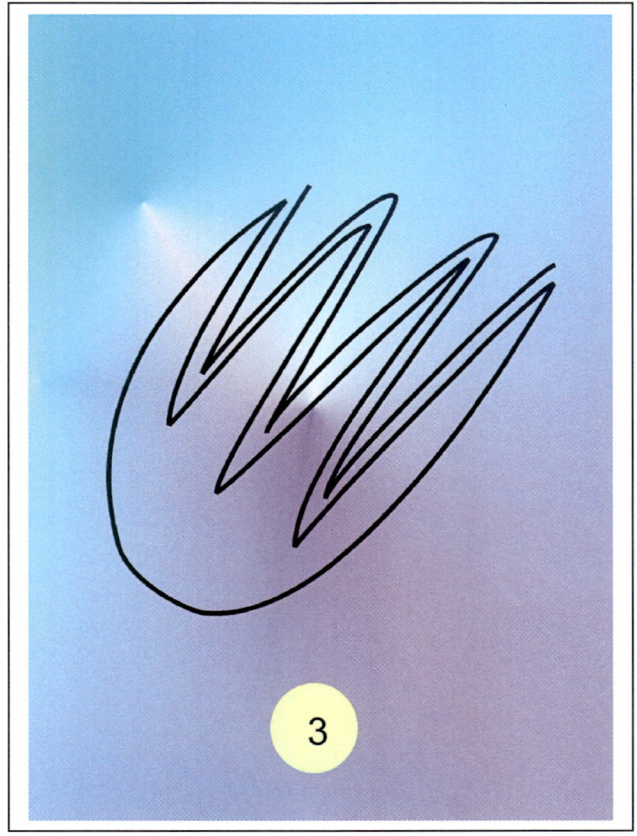

This person wishes these to remain in such a state for it gives them reasons not to follow their path in life.

19. This image shows the third ventricle in the brain with two tight restrictions in place to close down the third eye.

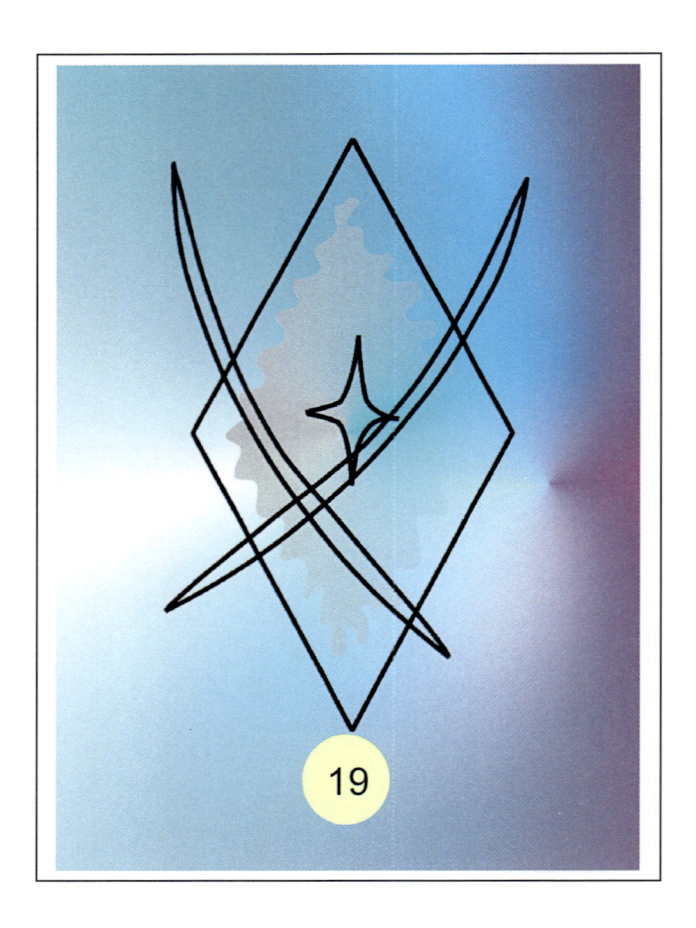

94. This image shows knots of self deception as the person chooses to feel depressed and to push the light far away.

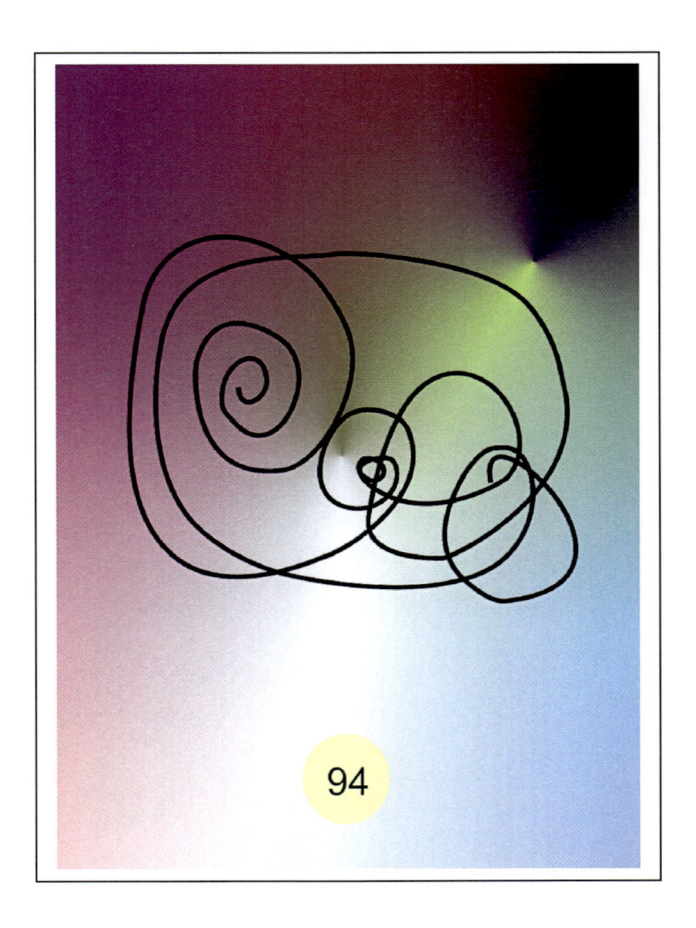

11. The Zodiac Angels for Capricorn 2

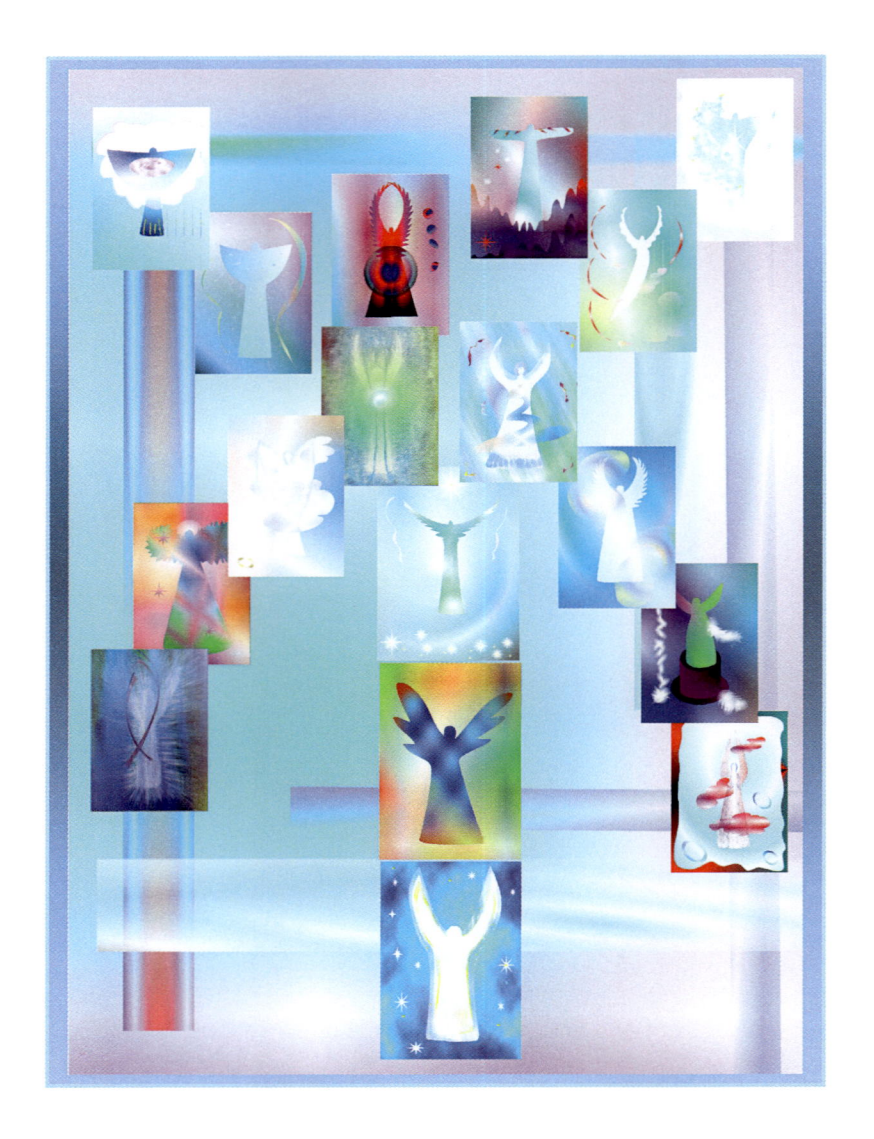

The Zodiac Angels for Capricorn 2

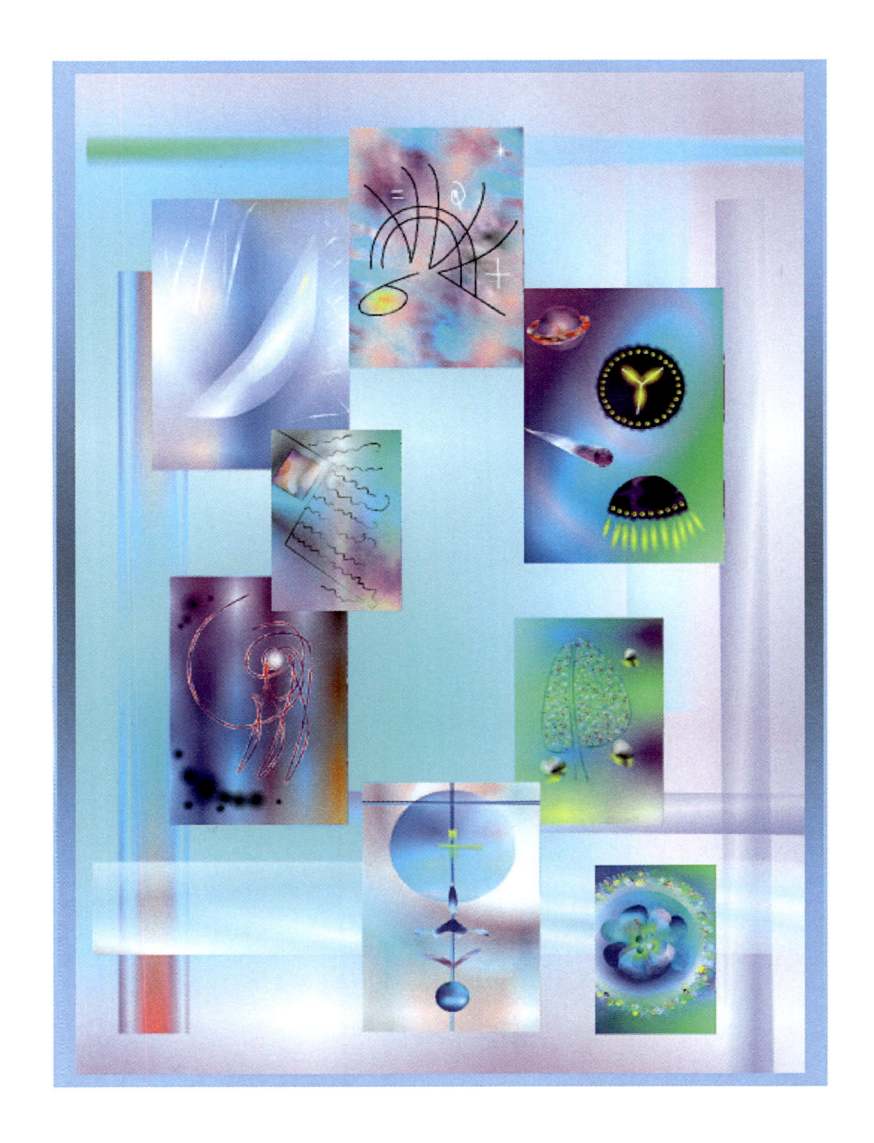

The Zodiac Art Images for Capricorn 2

The Zodiac Angels for Capricorn 2

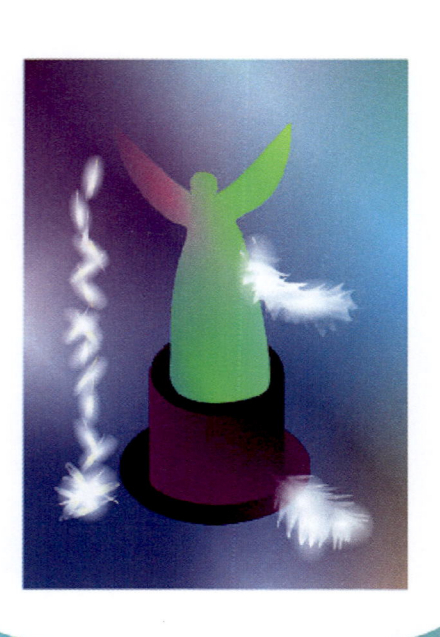

The Energy of the Larch

The energies of this time of the year are similar to the energies of the beautiful larch tree. The larch is a most unusual conifer. It has beautiful delicate pale green feathery leaves. It is unusual because it is deciduous and loses its delicate leaves in the autumn. There are large larch plantations across swathes of Canada and Russia as well as isolated specimens across the world in parks and gardens.

Its timber is very valuable as it is resistant to water and has been used for boat building for a long time. It is still used today for yachts, fencing and houses in Europe.

The Capricorn person, just like the larch tree is confident of being different and stands tall and proud. It can sense the truth of the world and is pleased to be a part of it.

'I am calmly able to say my piece'

The people born round the middle of Capricorn are the most focused of the Capricorns but their own lack of confidence or early knocks in life can obscure the view.

1.Azrael is one of the Alchemy Angels who have the power to transform our thoughts into nuggets of gold.

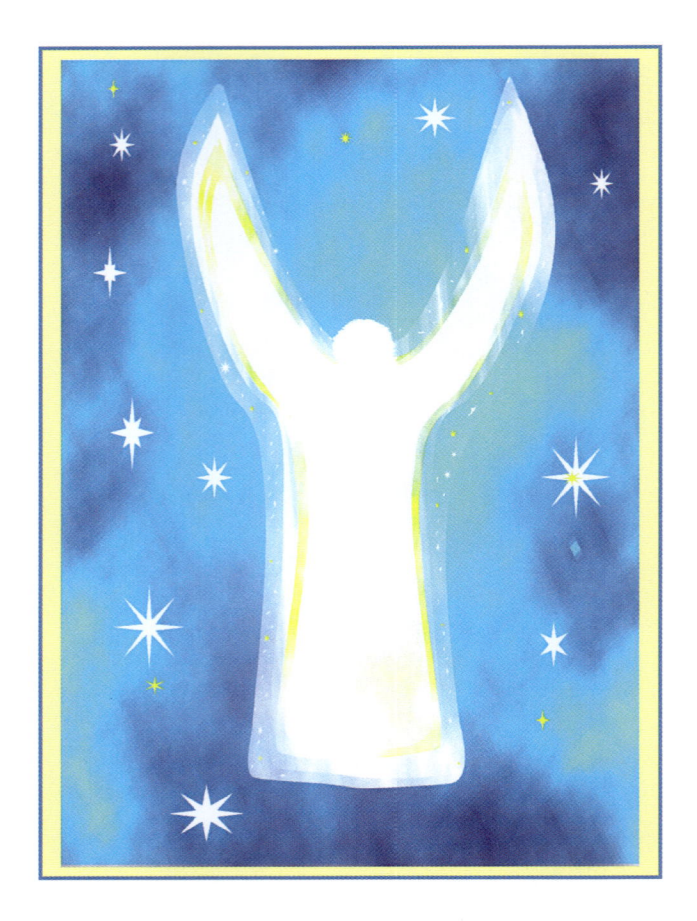

His message is

'Take a moment to reflect that you have already done so much that is truly amazing'.

2. **Amazine** is one of the Angels of Guidance. Amazine is a powerful Dark Angel to raise the spirits, lift the mood, and gives hope in the darkness of despair.

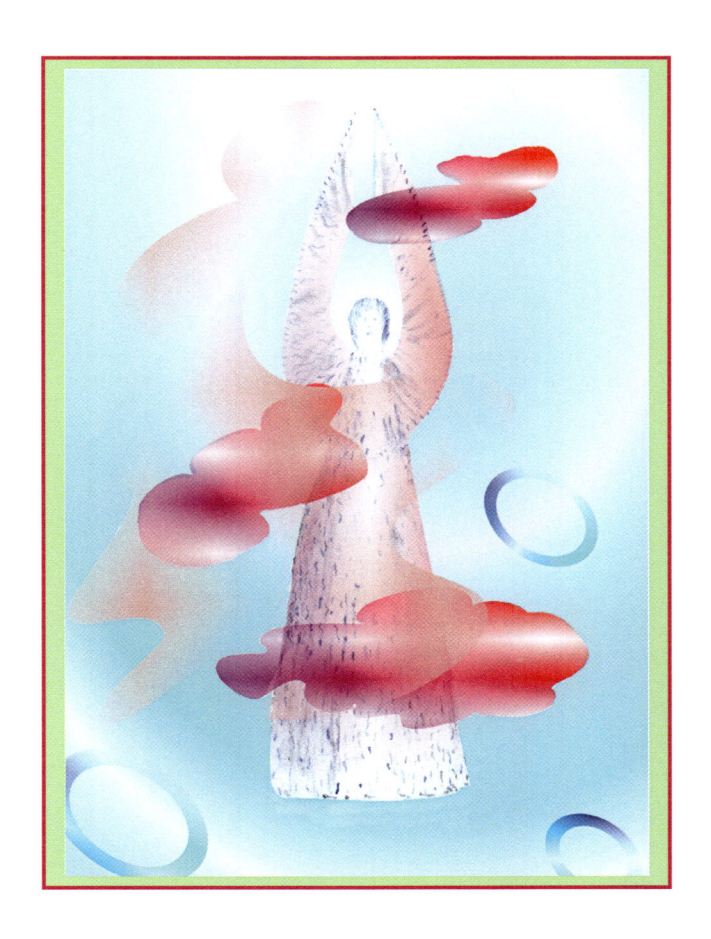

Amazine the Angel of Life

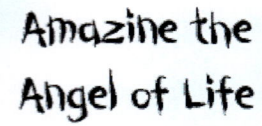

Amazine is around to raise the spirits of

anyone thinking that life is not worth living.

He can lift the mood and can give hope

in the darkness of despair.

Amazine restores faith in life itself and lights

up a path into the future.

With him around life is always

worth living and difficult times can always be healed.

3. Blasé is one of the Angels from the Matrix and the early days on the planet. She is for the quiet confident person standing up for their ideas-self assured and calm, even if others try to shout them down. There is a quiet surety about this person and they are often able to influence others in a quiet way.

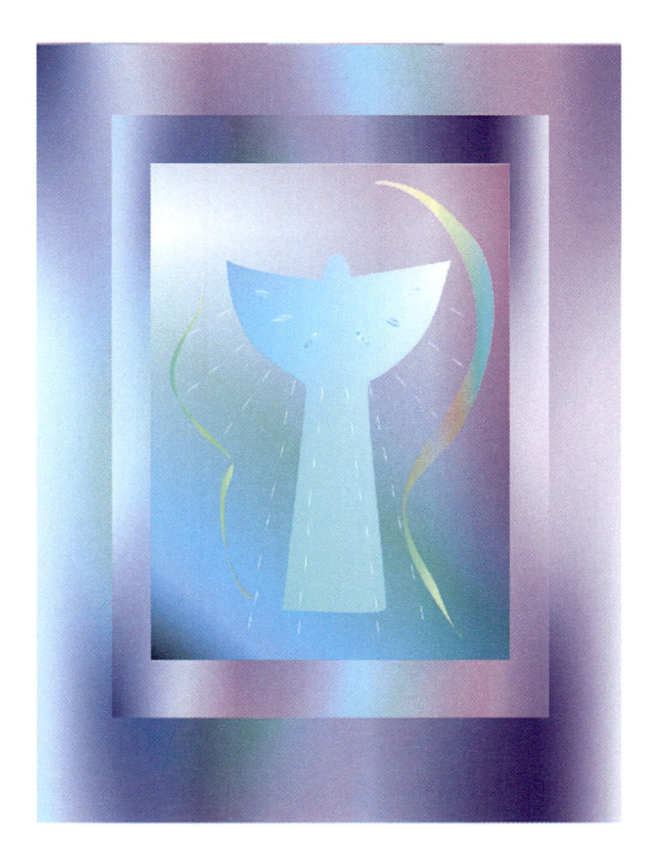

4. Bosalie is one of the Angels of the Challenges that have been chosen to be faced in this life. She has phenomenal power to help loosen the ties of past lives and to safely heal the memories within.

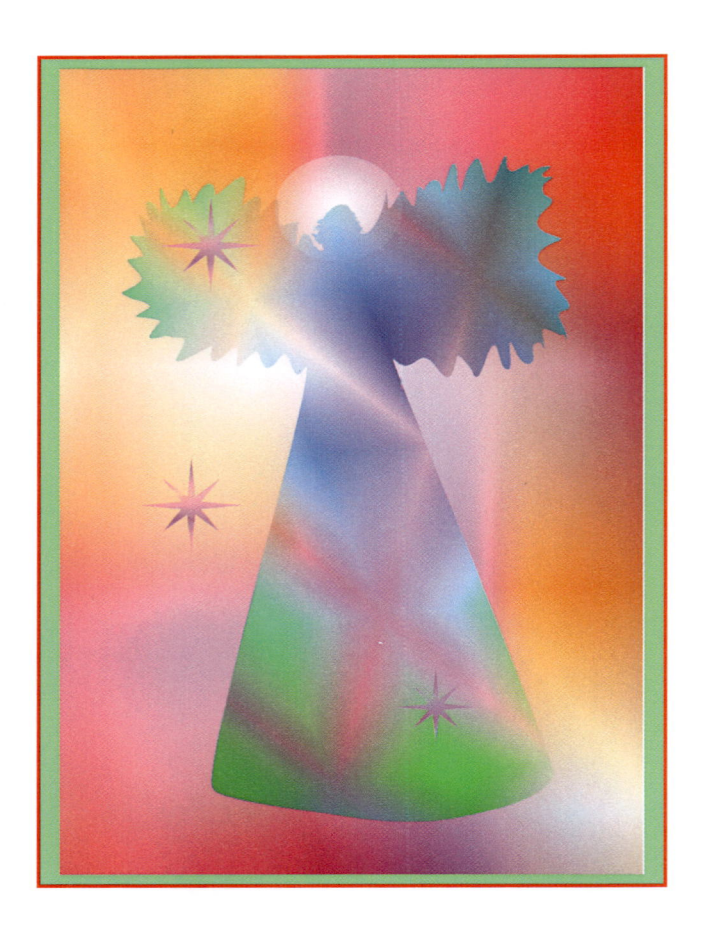

5. Celestina is one of the Alchemy Angels who have the power to transform our thoughts into nuggets of gold.

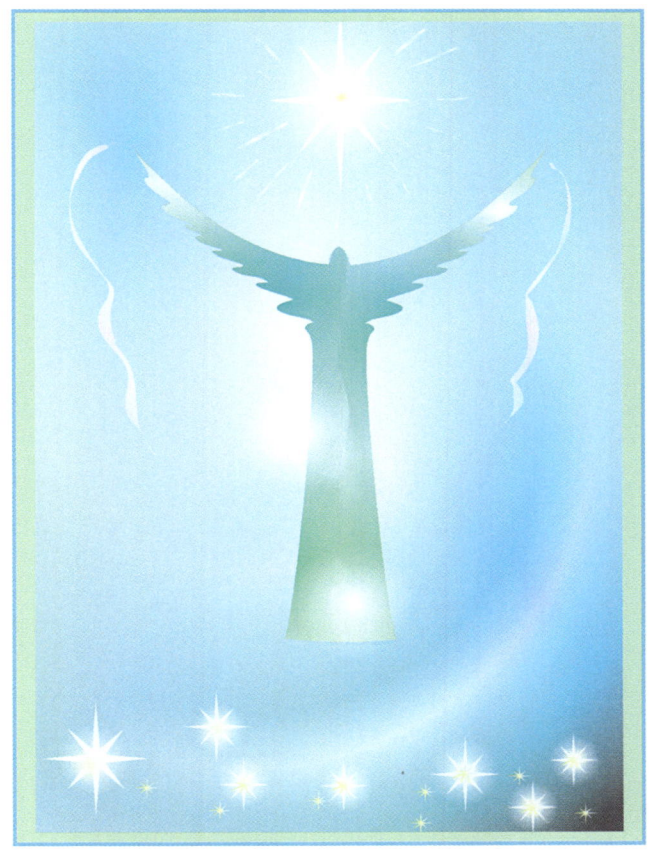

Her message is

'set yourself free to do whatever is necessary'

6. Confidence is an art image for the person who knows that confidence is their right but cannot find it .Confidence is like the feather, a feather of pure energy to inspire and guide and light the way. Trust the feather, climb aboard and float with it on an exciting voyage.

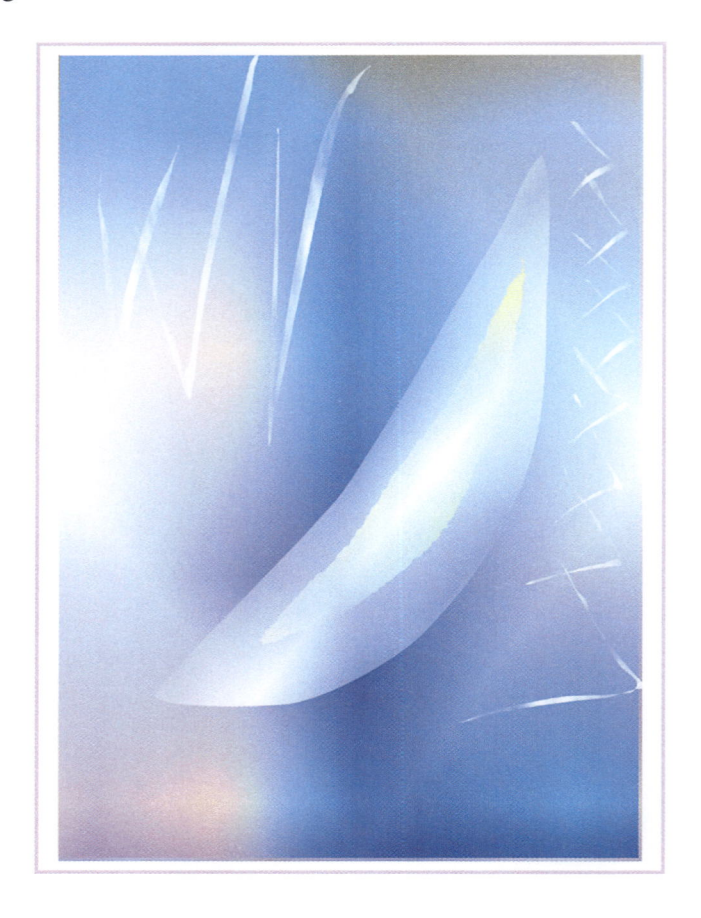

In so doing you can bring a light to brighten the lives of others.

7. Depression is one of the art images for the person who is still affected by the hatred from past lives. This hatred is held in place with sharp pins but it is safe to loosen these. Allow the angels into life and allow the angels to gently transmute the darkness into light for they have incredible power.

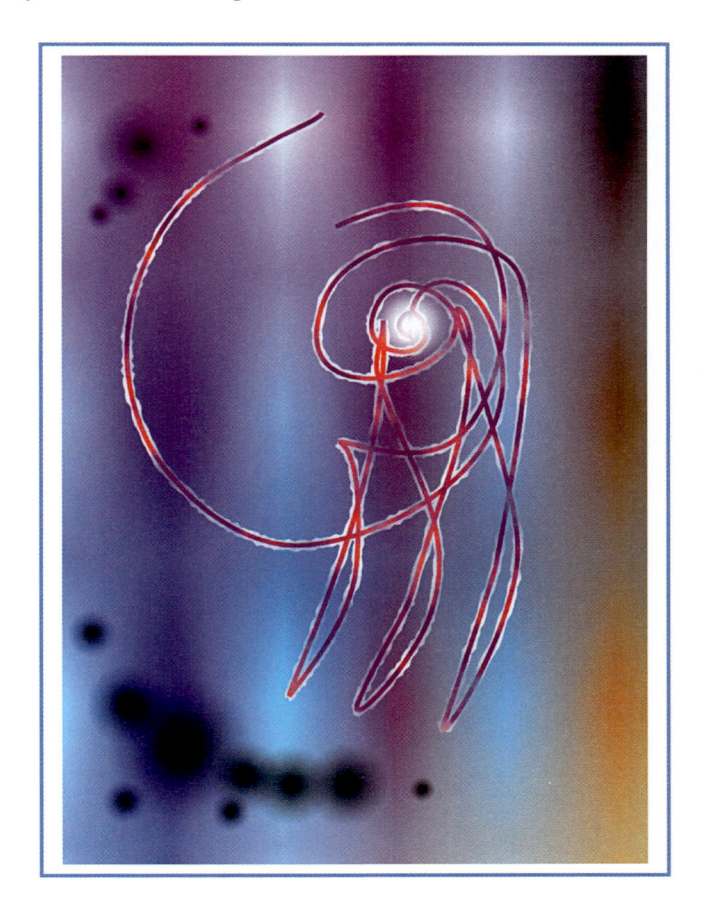

8. Elveen is the Angel of Imagination for the soul born between Jan 4th and Jan 7th. She is for the soul who imagines they are unable to ever speak their truth. She can help children succeed at school or perform on the stage and can help the soul at any age to speak their truth simply and with confidence.

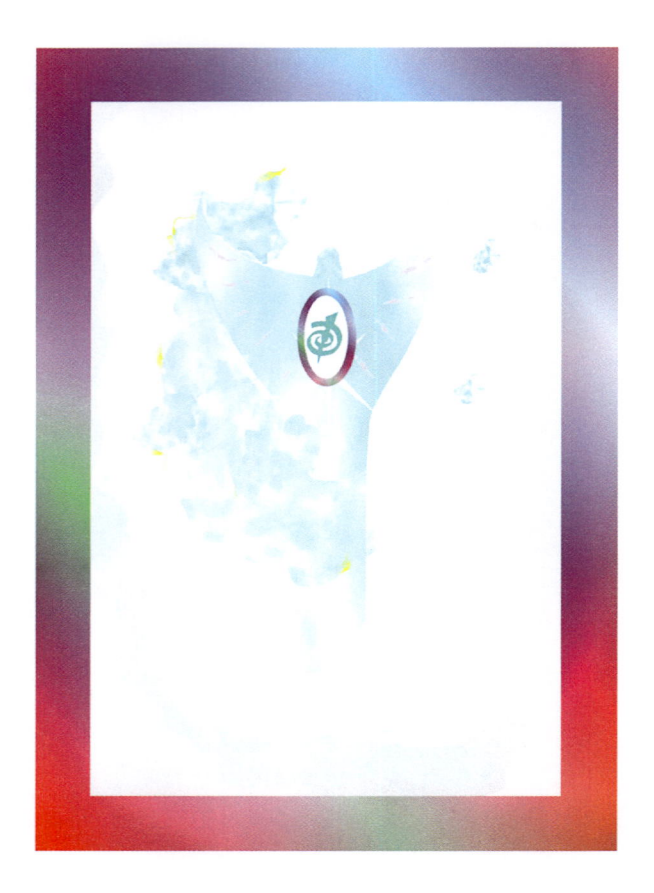

9.Frisson is a moonlight dream image for the person who has great knowledge and excitement inside them. Allow the bees to make their honey with your ideas for they can help many.

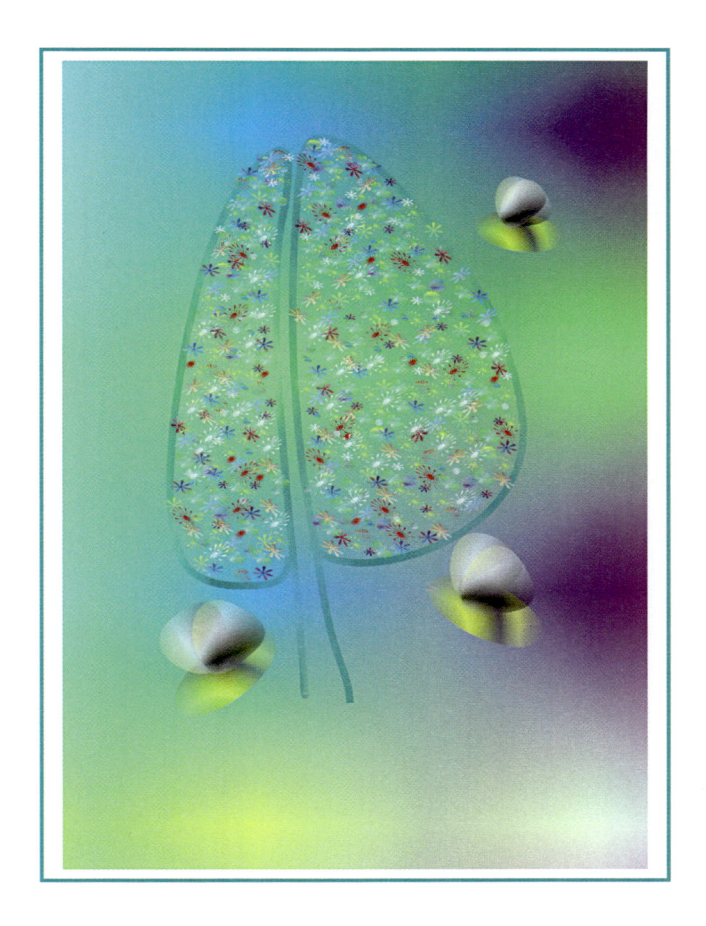

10. Hannah is one of the Earth Angels and gives clues to our problems. Hannah suggest that this soul may occasionally feel lacking in energy and unable to move. It is as if they are frozen with fear from the middle of a battle or a bad accident. Hannah is the angel to reach across troubled lands and to release old scars from the heart and the land.

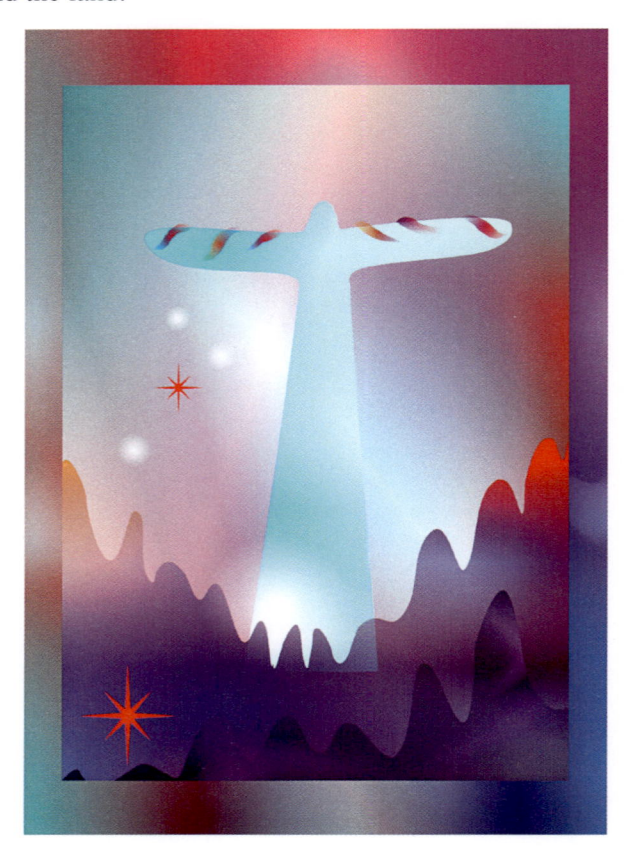

11. Harvey

Harvey is one of the powerful Angels of World Peace. He is the angel for the seer and the sensitive soul who needs protection as their gifts develop. There are many children who can see far beyond the horizon and into other dimensions. Others fear these visions and their lack of understanding closes down the spiritual side of the seer. It is a brave child with understanding parents who can retain and allow their psychic nature to grow and bloom. These children are different from most and need protection from Harvey as they often feel at 'odds' with the world and only want to be 'normal' like their friends.

Harvey has energies similar to homeopathic 'belladonna'. This is a very good remedy for children especially when the symptoms are acute red skin or throbbing headaches.

His message is

'believe in who you truly are for the truth is amazing'

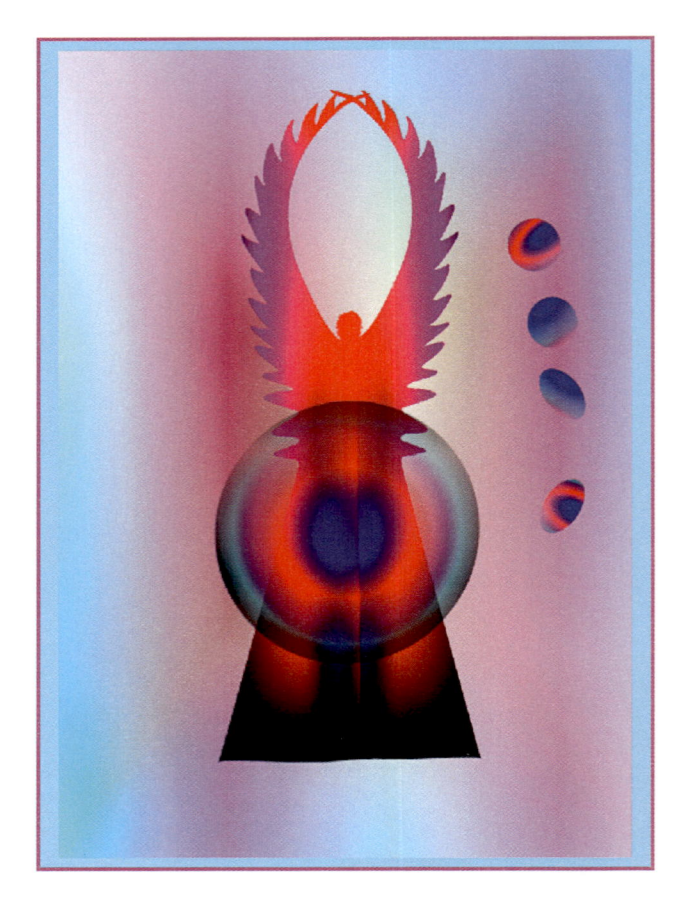

Harvey

12. Hashiele is one of the Rescue Angels for the person whose confidence was shattered by a parent or from the family. The memories from this still form a barrier around the heart. Hashiele allows these hurts to gently fade away and helps to find a new direction.

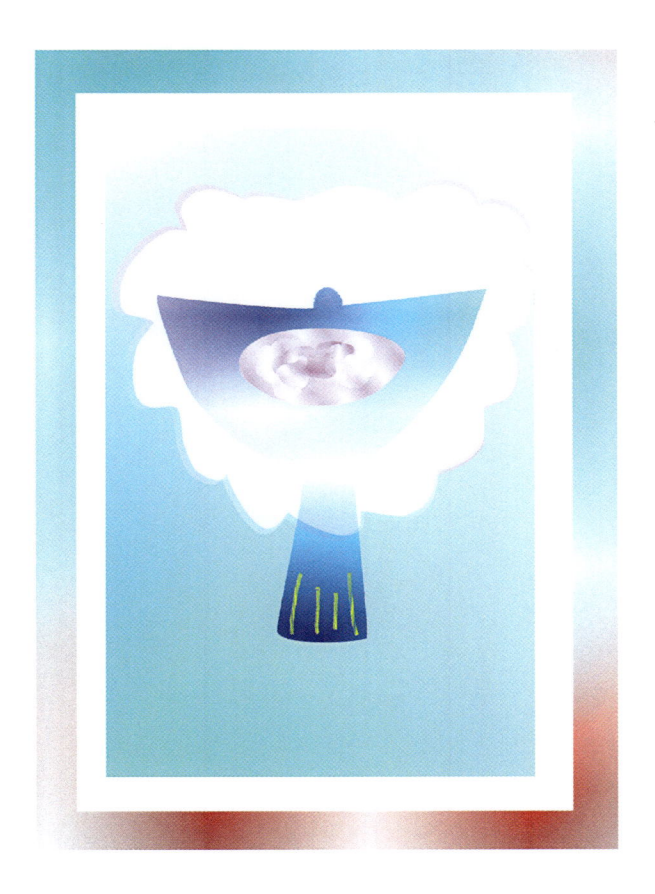

13. Myrriah is one of the Angels of Innocence and of childhood days when life seemed easier and the world new and exciting.

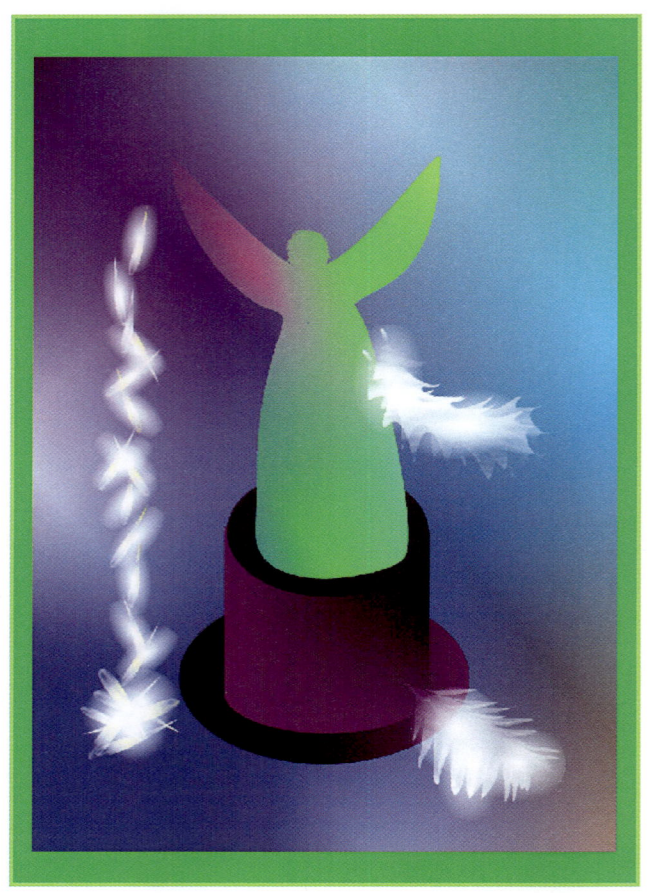

These are the angels of sharing with friends and the sheer enjoyment of the simple things in life such as emerging from a top hat with feathers flying and settling in patterns. Allow these angels to bring fun and magic back into your life.

14.Opportunity is an art image for the person who has the courage to follow the path. There will be small steps and large leaps until the end is in sight. The path is always so and may even have steps which feel as if they take us backward. Every step is important and from every step the person can learn so much. Allow yourself to view such apparent backward steps in a different way.

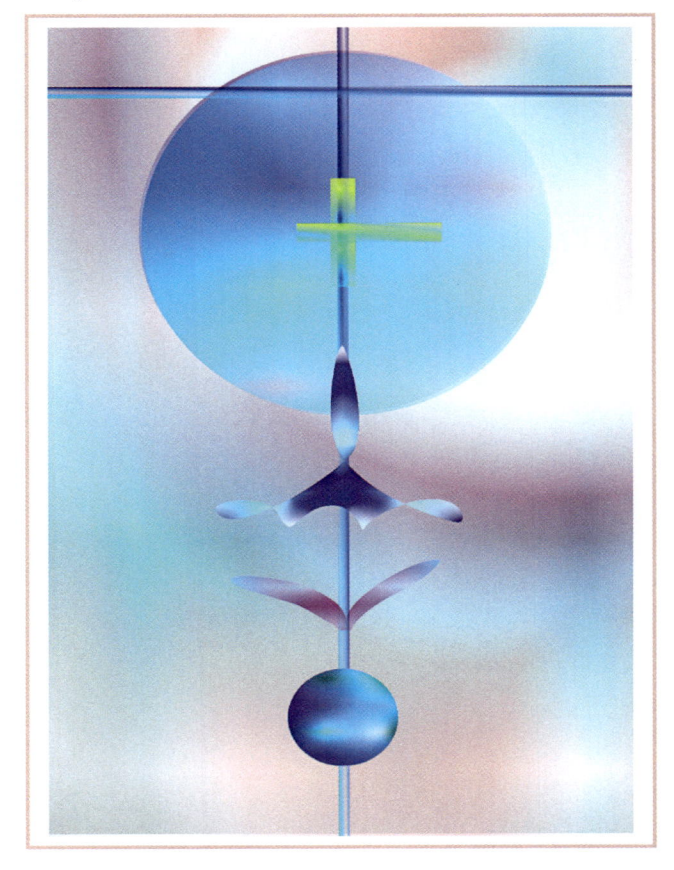

15. Papise is the Angel of Imagination for the soul born between Jan 1st and Jan 3rd. This soul feels that they want to run away from life and responsibilities. Life seems difficult why can they not just dream and be themselves. This is the imagination talking for this Capricorn person is very capable and is able to bring a balance into their life where there is time for their own needs.

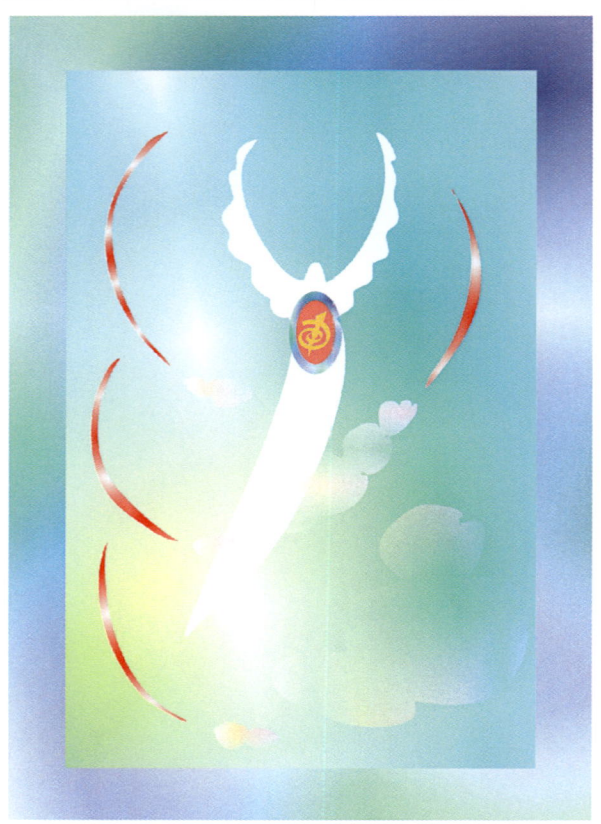

16. Persistence is a moonlight dream image for the soul who tries to run away from problems. By doing so they are not true to themselves and the problems will continually lurk in the back of the mind. This soul needs to face the truth for eternal peace and innermost serenity. With the angels around the truth is far easier to face.

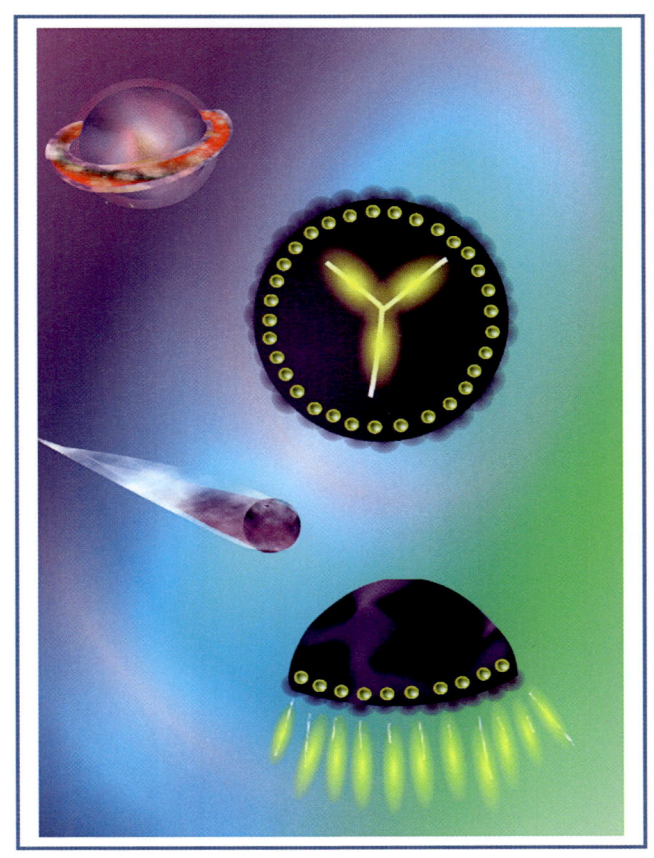

17. Porterie is one of the Angels of the Shifting Sands who can help to transform our lives if we so desire. Deep within this person are many fears which Porterie can gently blow away with a sweep of her wings if you ask her to help.

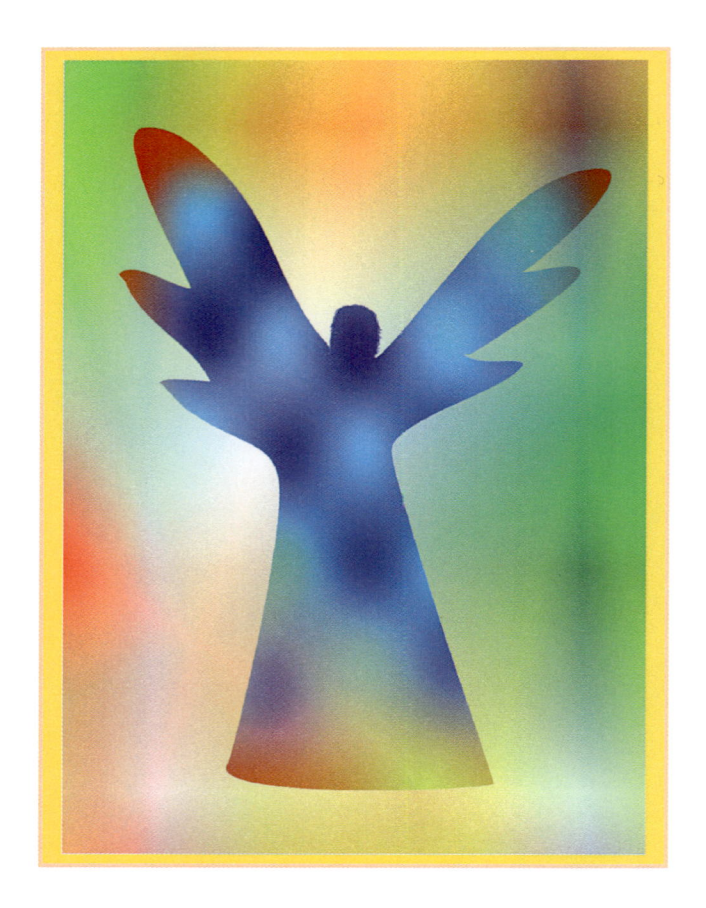

18. Rachel is the Angel of Imagination for the soul born between Jan 8th and Jan 10th. This angel is for the soul who has great capabilities and can lead others. They may not have been encouraged in early life and so doubt their own abilities. You have amazing powers so use these for yourself, family and friends.

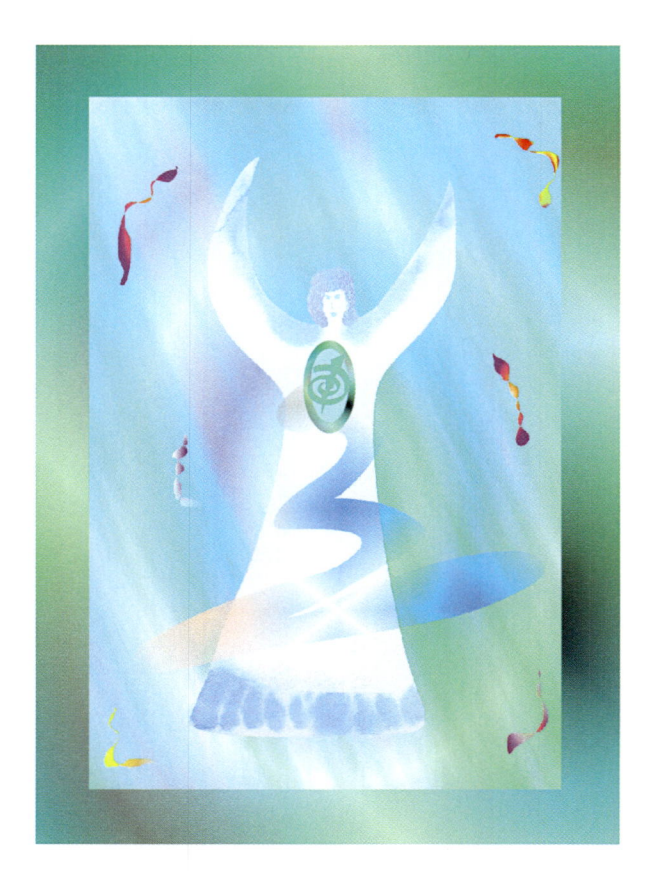

19. Shadowy is an enchantment image for the soul who fears their shadow side. On looking into the depths of the well or their own soul they sense unease for no reason. This is often due to many emotions being suppressed rather than faced with calm.

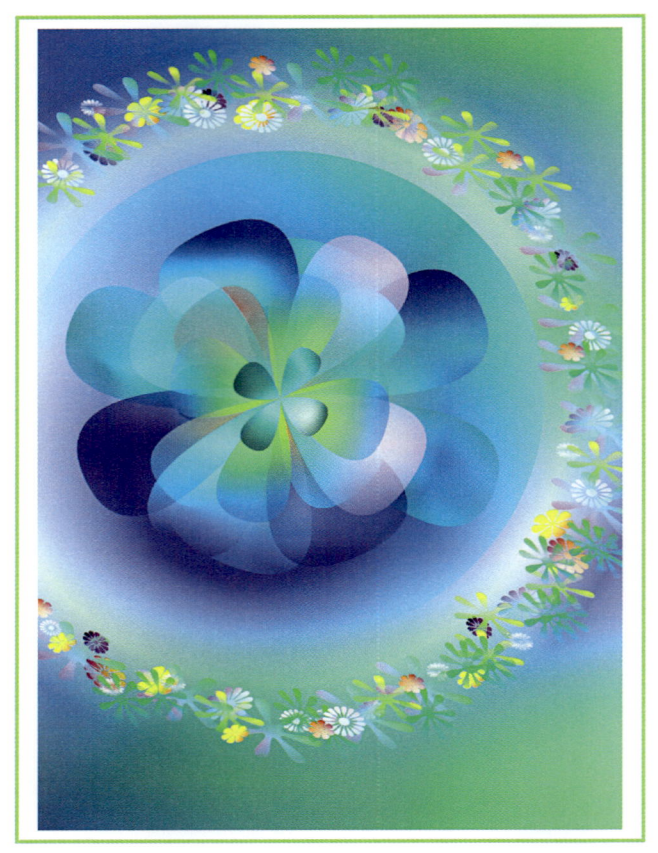

Allow the beauty of this flower to lessen the unease and instil a sense of calm and peace.

20. Shyness is a harmony image for the person who envies others their ease of speaking out or being the centre of attention. This person feels unwanted and tries to hide behind others. The box of shyness can gently be opened by the angels and this can allow the effervescence of this character to slowly emerge into the light.

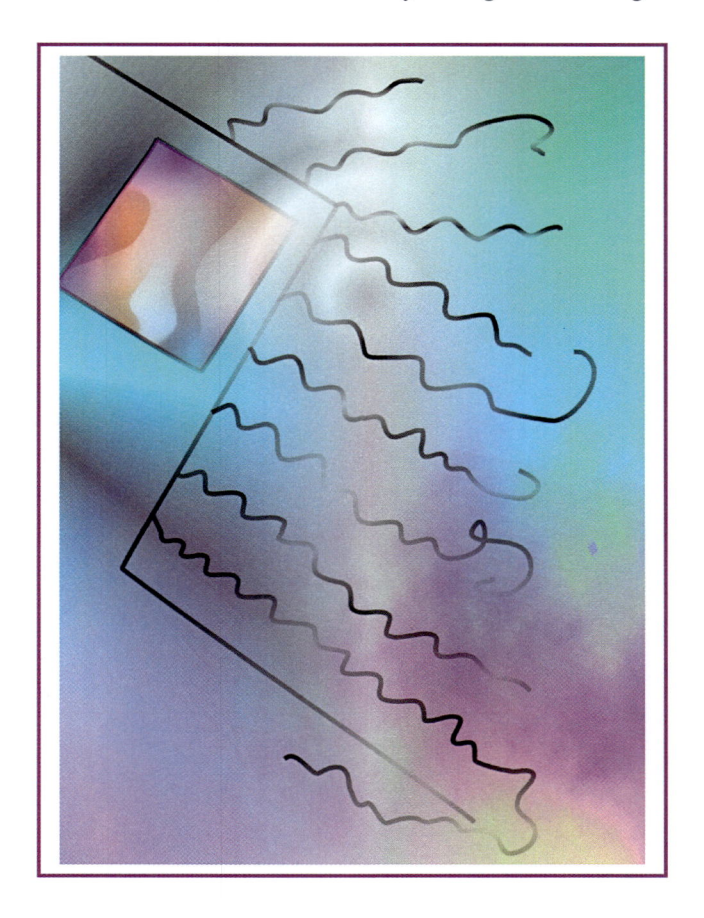

21. Tamsie is one of the Angels at the end of the Rainbow where the pot of gold can be found. This soul feels as if they are hidden and unable to get their message and personality across to others. let Tamsie help along the journey as obstacles can be lessened and the voice can begin to get out to others.

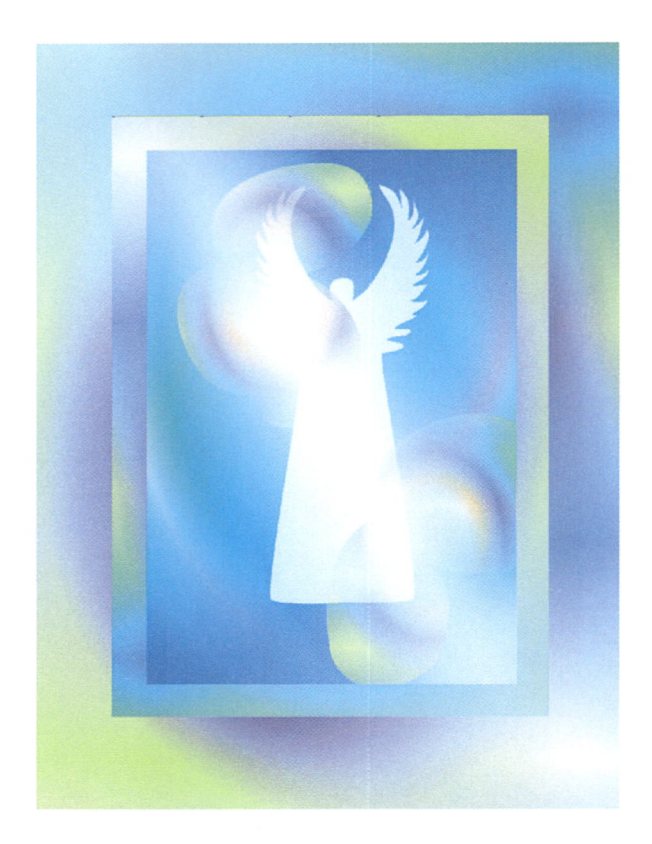

22. Tarquille is one of the Angels of Guidance. The single ring symbolises a break from someone in the past to set both people free to move forward. He could also symbolise that in order to be free to move on it is important to release the need for marriage and vows as a strong desire for anything can work to prevent its outcome.

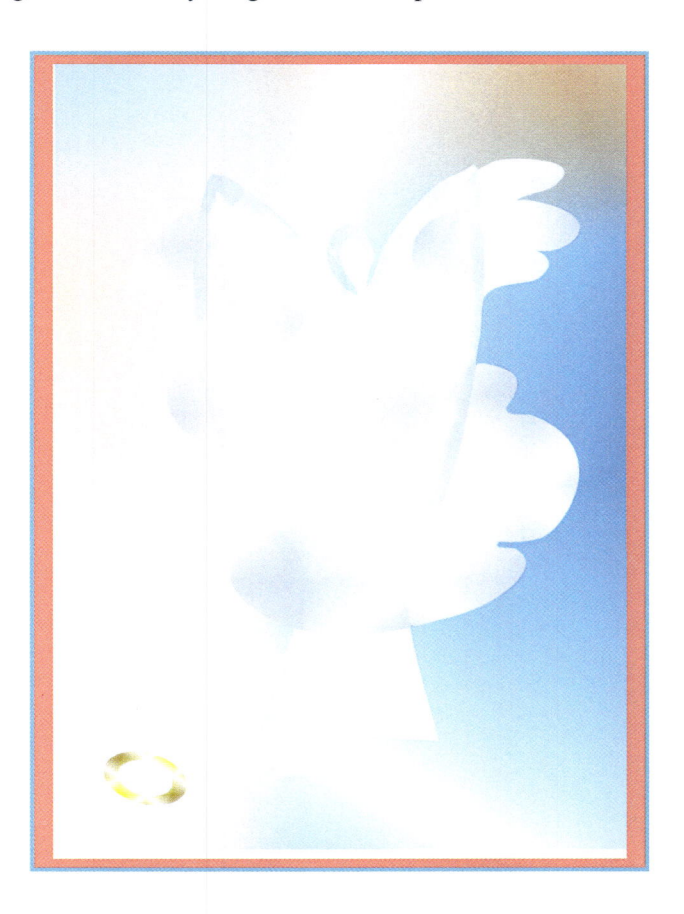

Tarquille the Angel of Freedom

Tarquille can help peeople be released from

old vows made in the past.

He helps people move on and start again.

The single gold ring symbolises a fresh start

and a bright future.

23. Visionary is a harmony image for the person who is truly visionary . They have amazing ideas which can inspire others from stories to music or ways of being. Trust your knowing and use your ideas to invent or build a better world for others.

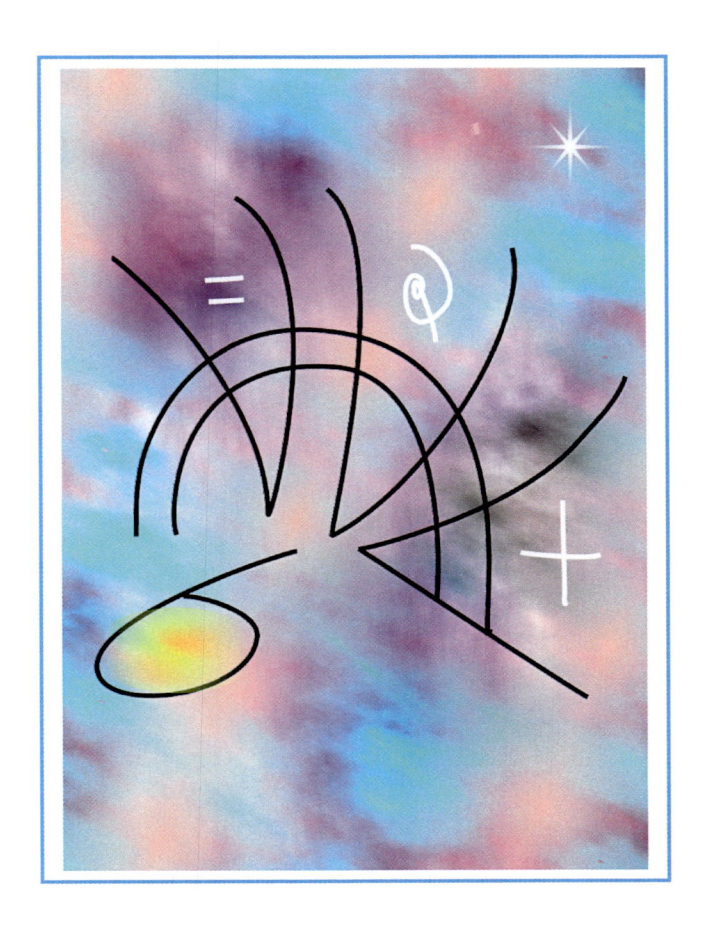

Images of Excitement

23. There are many gossamer strands linking you to past lives where hurts have played a big part in life. You do not need to continue to carry these for they bear no relationship to your life today.

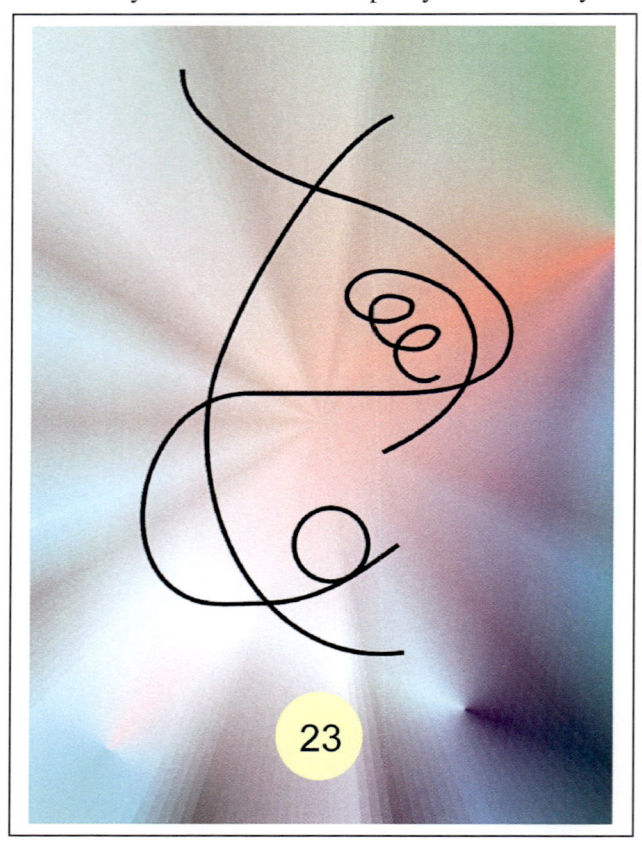

40. This image is for the person who imagines many hooks around their spine and within the tight muscles of the back. Sit quietly and imagine theses straightening for they are no longer needed.

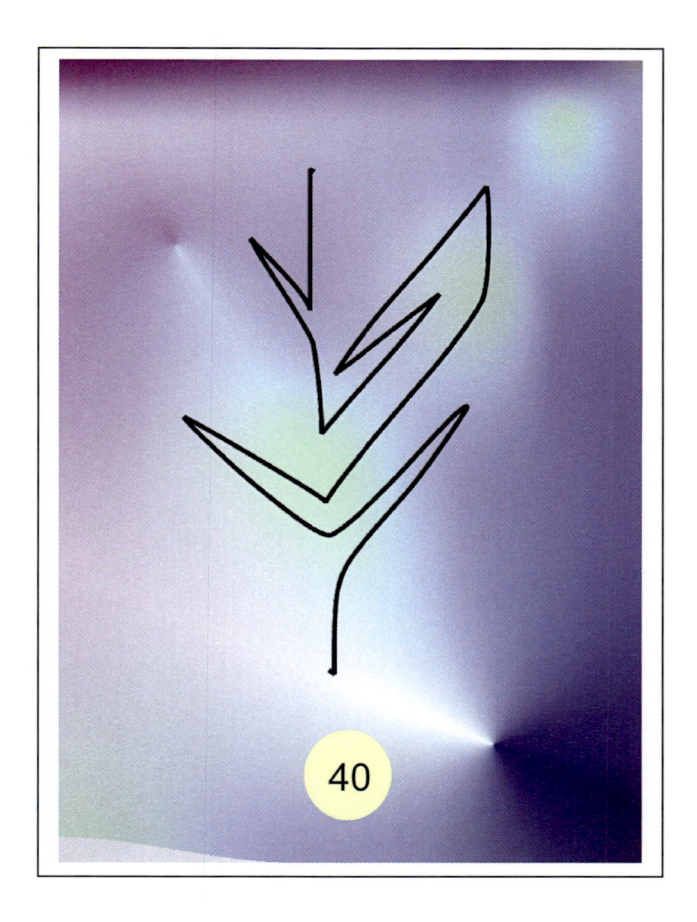

104. This image contains the hook of despair as the person imagines that life can never alter. It can especially with theses angels in your life.

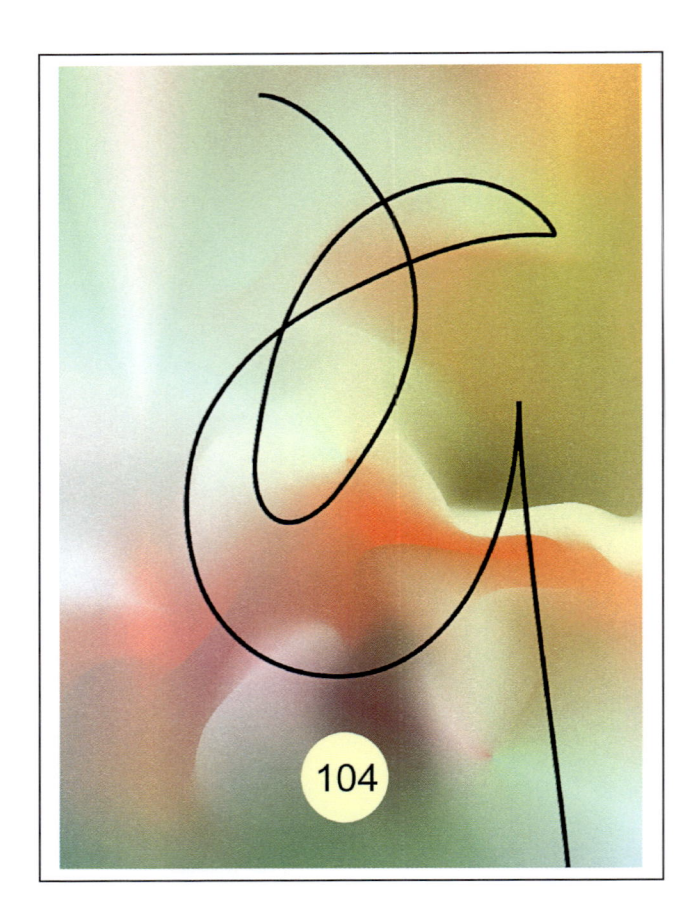

12. The Zodiac Angels for Capricorn 3

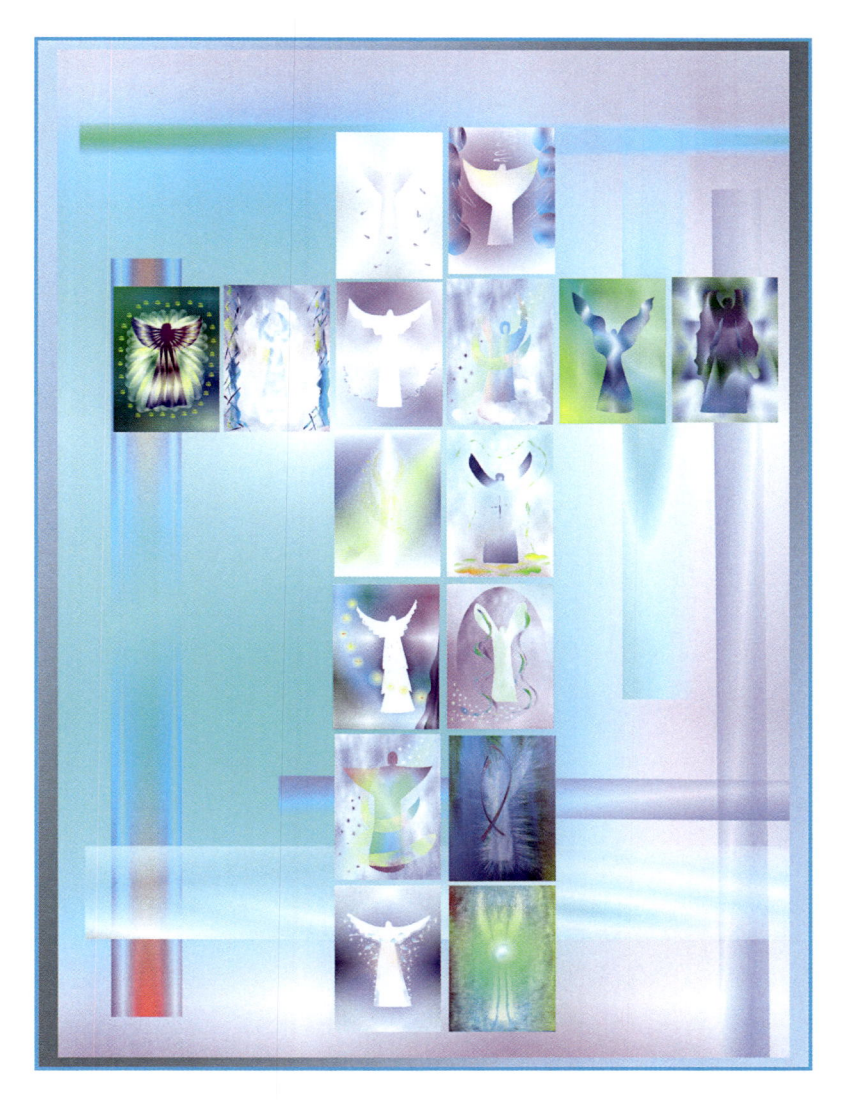

The Zodiac Angels for Capricorn 3

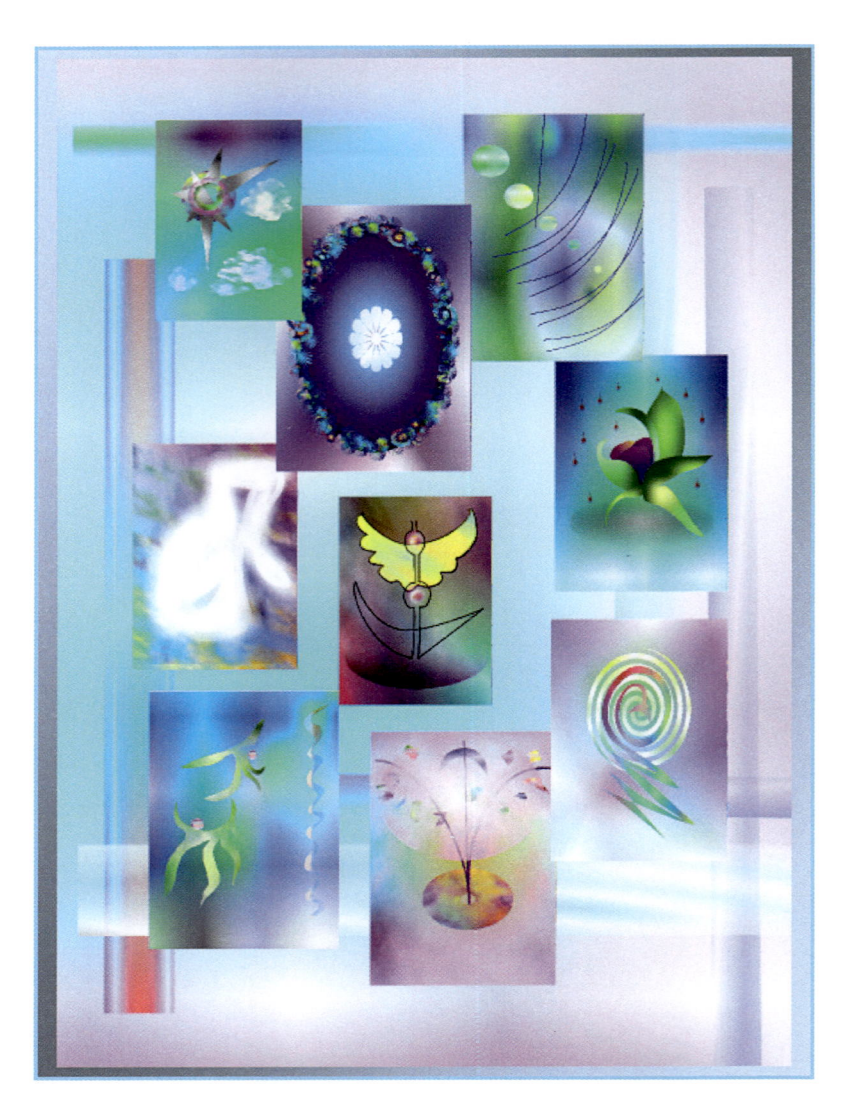

The Zodiac Art Images for Capricorn 3

The Zodiac Angels for Capricorn 3

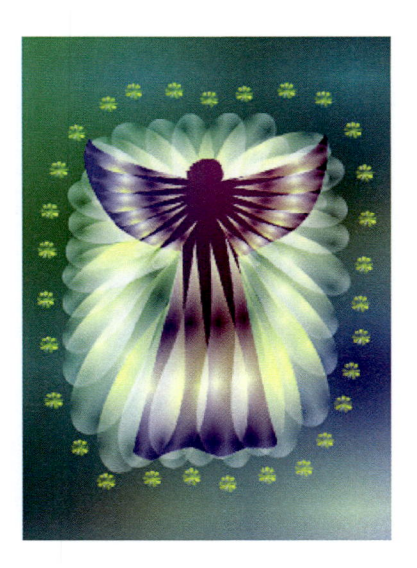

The Energy of the Gentian

The gentian is a hardy biennial plant which grows on poor, acidic soils often on dry hills, cliffs or sand dunes. It produces vibrant tubular flowers of blue, crimson or purple. The gentian seeds are thrown to the winds and most fail to thrive. If lucky, a seed begins to germinate in the right conditions. The high mortality rate for the seeds, give rise to feelings of abandonment by their parents very early on in life. Many seeds begin to grow but a change in weather conditions can easily halt them before their prime as they wither and die in splendid isolation. The gentian person, like the plant, feels a lack of encouragement and respect, particularly from a father figure. This feeling could also arise from a parent who is over protective and does not encourage their child to reach high. This makes it difficult to find the confidence to go far out into the world, to reach for the top and to mark our own mark. Without this early encouragement the gentian soul loses sight of who they are they can become depressed and despondent. They stubbornly find it difficult to believe that it is their own lack of faith and negative attitudes which holds them back. The gentian soul either feels abandoned by their parents or has parents who are over protective and does not encourage their child to reach far. This makes it difficult to find the confidence the highest and to mark our own mark.

'no task is too great because I believe'

1. Balance is an art image for the soul who needs balance in life. As we drift in the oceans of life we are pearls among the sea delicately trying to find a balance in all things. This person is easily thrown out of balance as their right brain tends to be blocked.

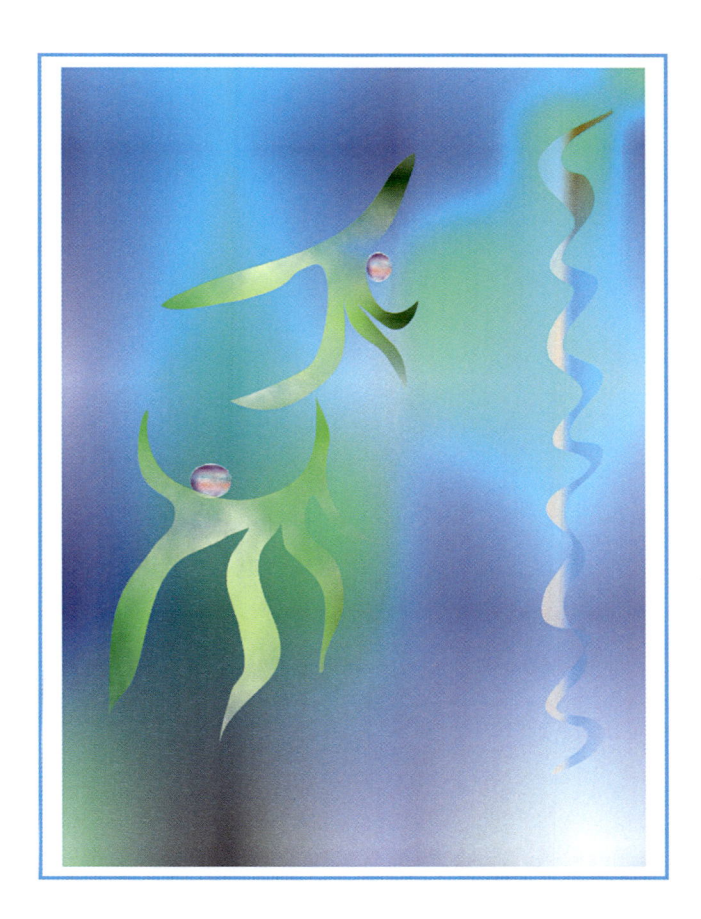

2. Disdain is a harmony image for the soul who has high ideals and feels others should live their life in the same way. This person often feels superior to others who they see as harming their bodies as with smoking or eating junk food. Everyone learns at their own pace in lie so have empathy for others.

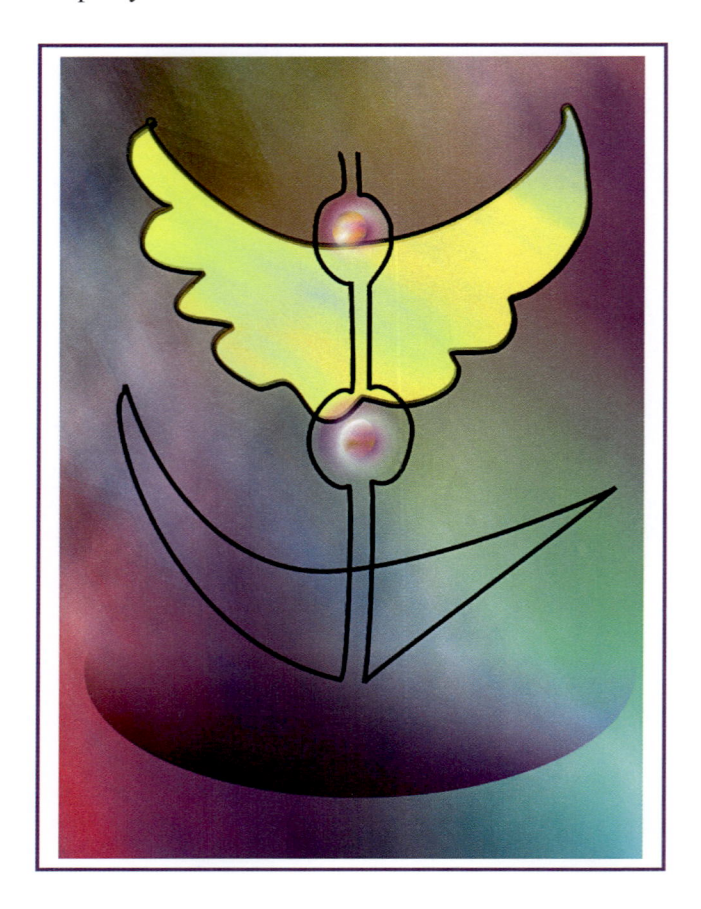

3. Dorang is one of the Earth Angels who give clues over problems which hold us back. This angel can, with a sweep of her wings organise others and loves doing so. They are very good at charity work but in their eagerness to achieve they sometimes alienate others with their zeal and determination.

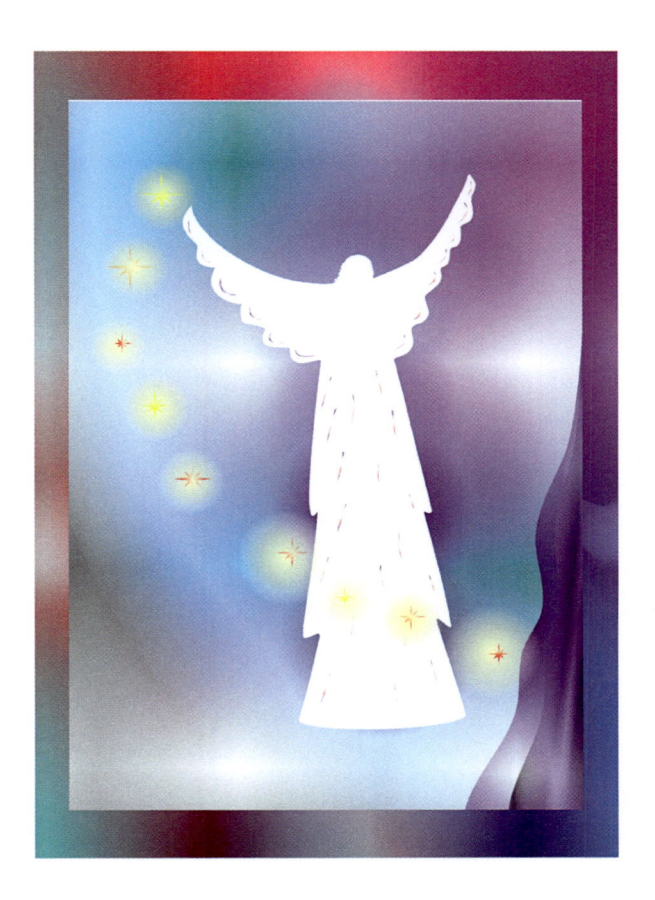

4. Effervescent is an ancestral image for the person who knows the great joy from giving to others as food, money or overseas aid. This soul believes they always have to be the one in control. If they can let go of this need then the inner fountain of joy and spiritual wealth erupts in full and the funfair ride can be truly enjoyed.

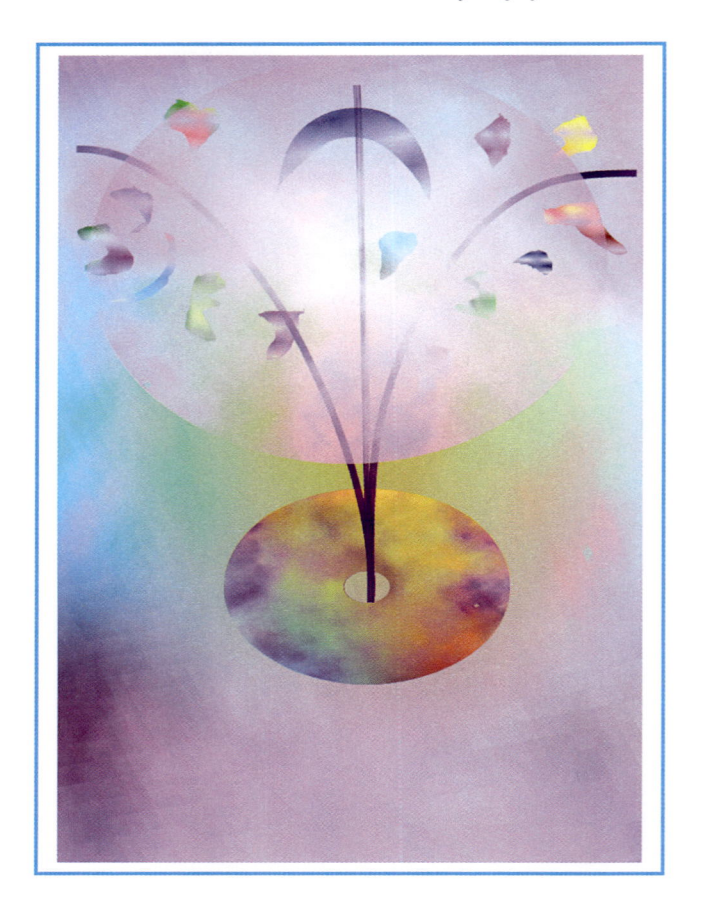

Their emotions can reach out to touch others in the same way as their gifts do, reaching a powerful crescendo of endless love.

5. Ego is an art image for the person who has an overactive left side of their brain ignoring the intuitive right side. They also feel the need to be in control of others and to dominate their lives.

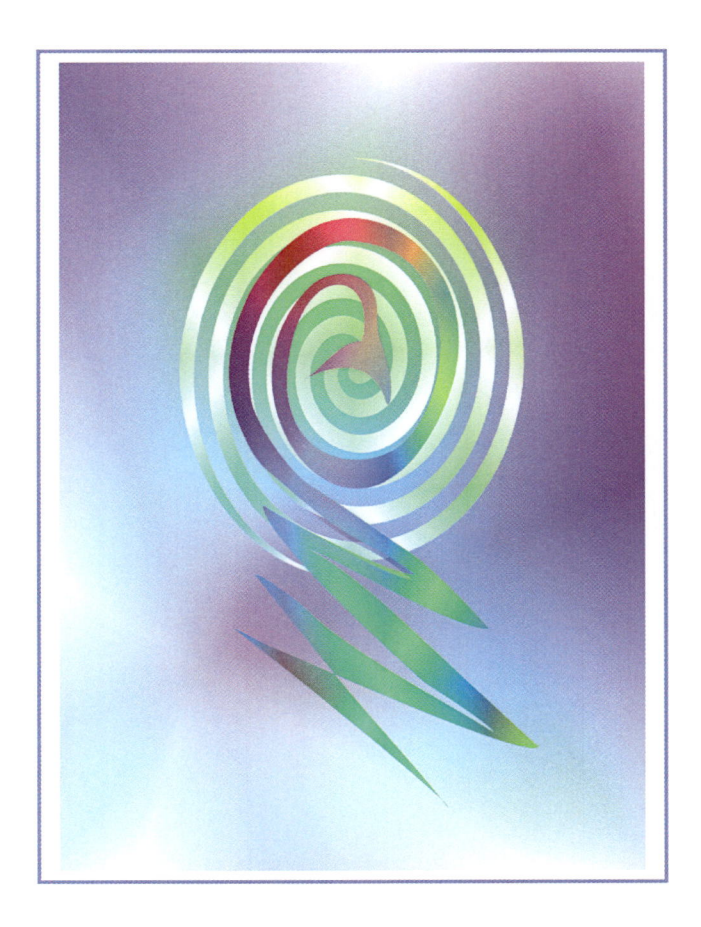

6. Folio is one of the Angels of Enlightenment and is the angel of ermine and the of the crown. Folio can help us to know the truth of the world through the gift of clairsentience and of just knowing.

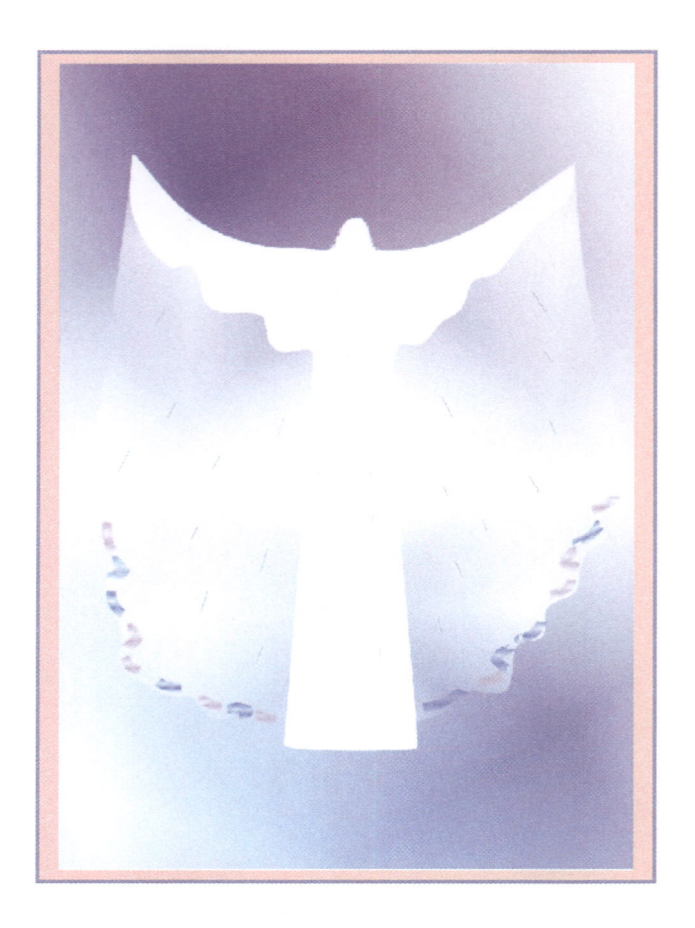

7. Gabriel is one of the Archangels of Guidance. He is a beacon, the Archangel to welcome someone home on the spiritual plane as they are following long time dreams. He appears for enlightened souls who are truly illuminated with the spiritual glow. The stars within the swathe are all the connections within the spiritual family and welcome the person back fully into the fold of similar souls.

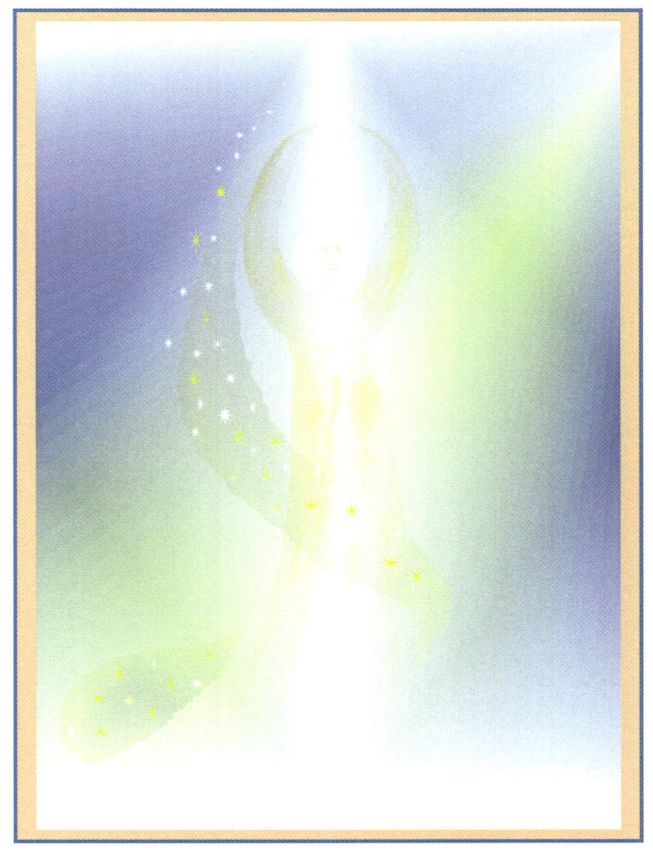

Once Gabriel has entered lives then guidance comes fast along with intuition and fulfilling potential at the highest level.

Gabriel the Homecoming Angel

Gabriel is a beacon, the archangel to welcome someone

home on the spiritual plane as they follow

their long time dreams.

The stars are all connections with the spiritual

family and welcome the person back

into their spiritual family.

After Gabriel enters lives then

changes occur and life is never the same again.

8. Illious is one of the Angels of the Matrix and of the early days on the planet. She is the angel of meditation. She shows the peace, harmony and love to be found within the soul as the inner light is reached. This is the absolute stillness that can be found during meditation with a free flowing imagination finding hidden sparks and gems to inspire life.

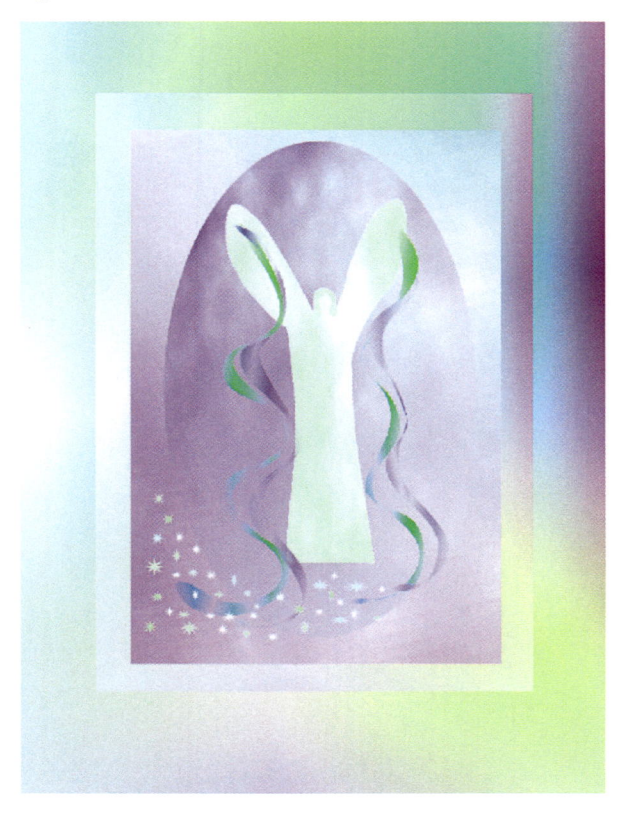

This person rarely meditates for they fear the loss of control.

9. Innocence is an ancestral image for the soul who feels shocked by some incident in their past. This shock can remain deep inside as a numbness for decades. With these angels around a gentle love can begin to infuse the body and the soul and lightens the load.

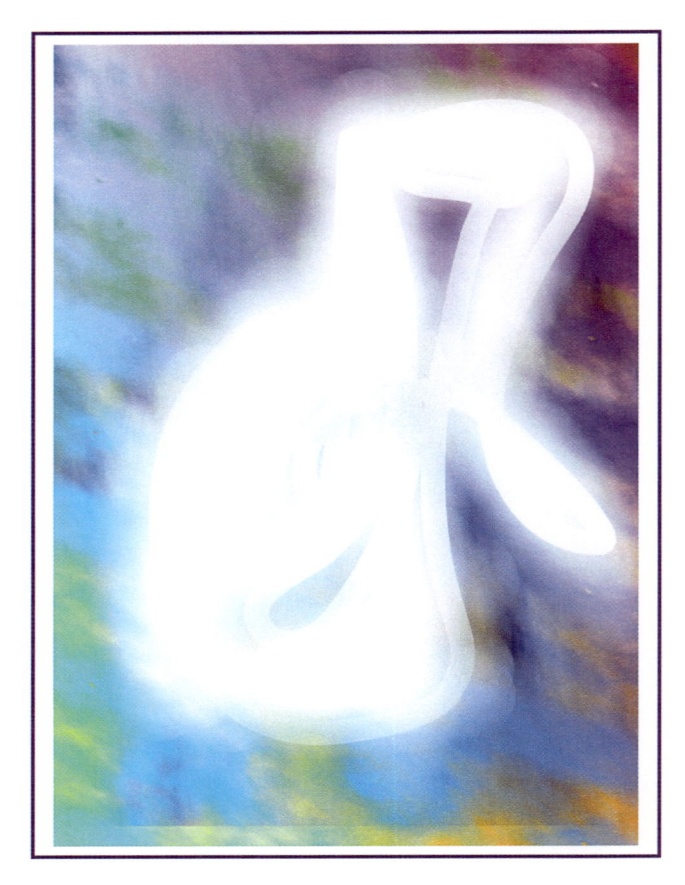

Without help this shock can tighten many muscles causing pains for years.

10.Lividious is one of the Angels of the Challenges that have been chosen to be faced in this lifetime. Her incredible wings can delve deeply into the body to release fears which only prevent the person coming into their own.

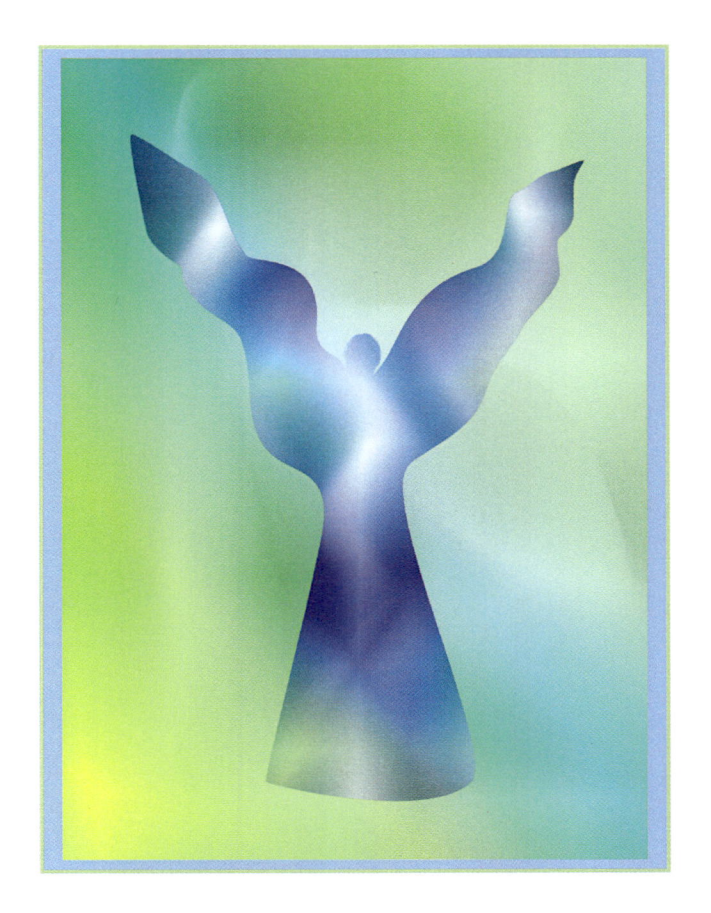

11. Longevity is a moonlight dream image for the person who has lived many lives to the full. Even so they are still worthy of feeling clear sparkling drops of rain not blood splattered ones from battles or trauma.

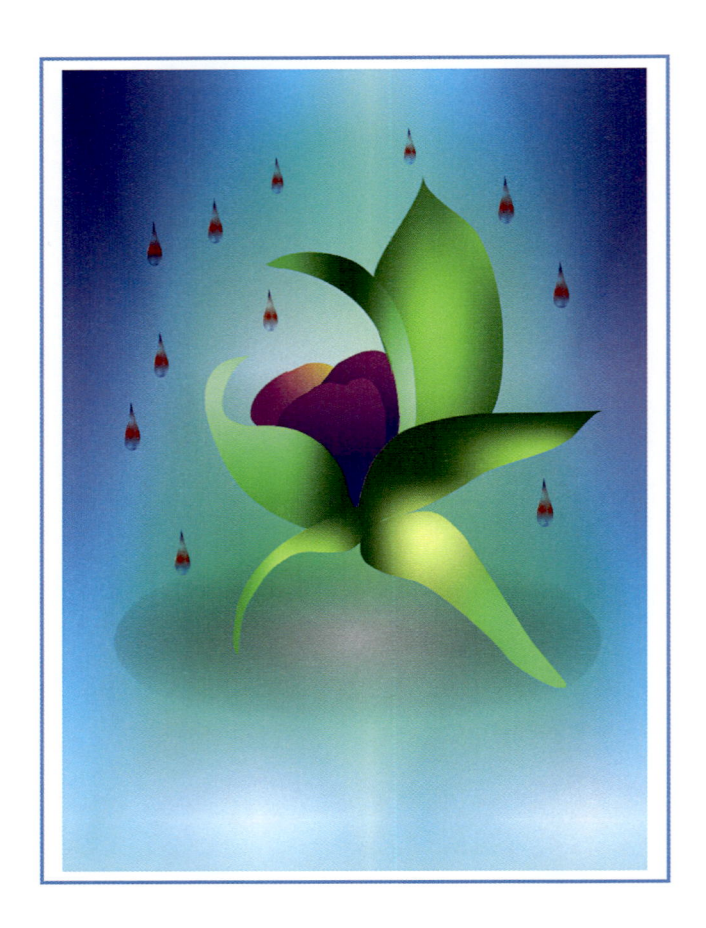

12.Mackie is one of the Angels of the Shifting Sands who can help us to change our lives if we wish. She can help calm to return after more traumatic lives or the storms of earlier days. Let her work her magic.

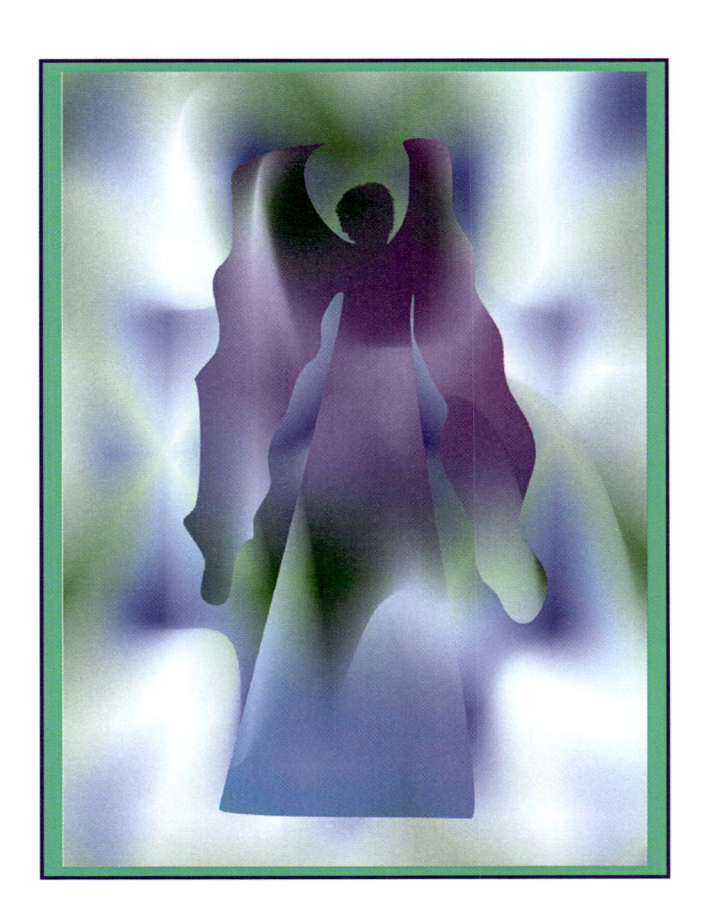

13. Persepio is one of the Angels of Rescue for the soul who feels fears creeping into their lives and into their heart, bringing with them a black dog mood. With Persepio around the fears can be lightened from within and be transformed into a gentle joy.

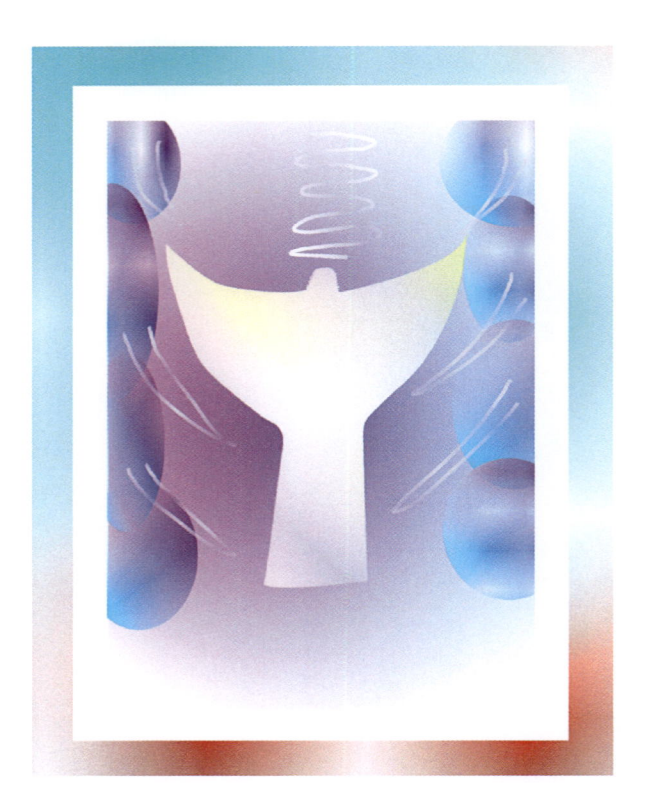

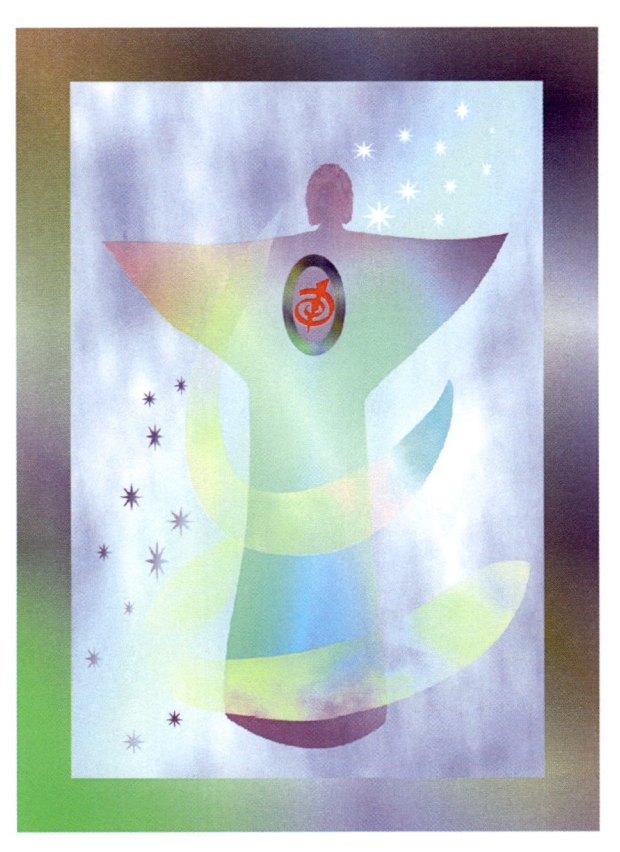

14.Rainbow is the Angel of the Imagination for the soul born between Jan 18th and Jan 20th. This soul fears the unseen world of the spirits. At times they can sense this world but with clairsentience they cannot easily see or hear, they feel fear. Rainbow is surrounded by stars as she transmutes your fears into sparks to light the fire in the soul.

15. Raziel is the Angel of the Imagination for the soul born between Jan 11th and Jan 13th. This angel appears for the soul who feels that they have been repeating patterns in life after life and are unable to see a different outcome. With these angels come a fresh eye and a fresh impetus and change is inevitable.

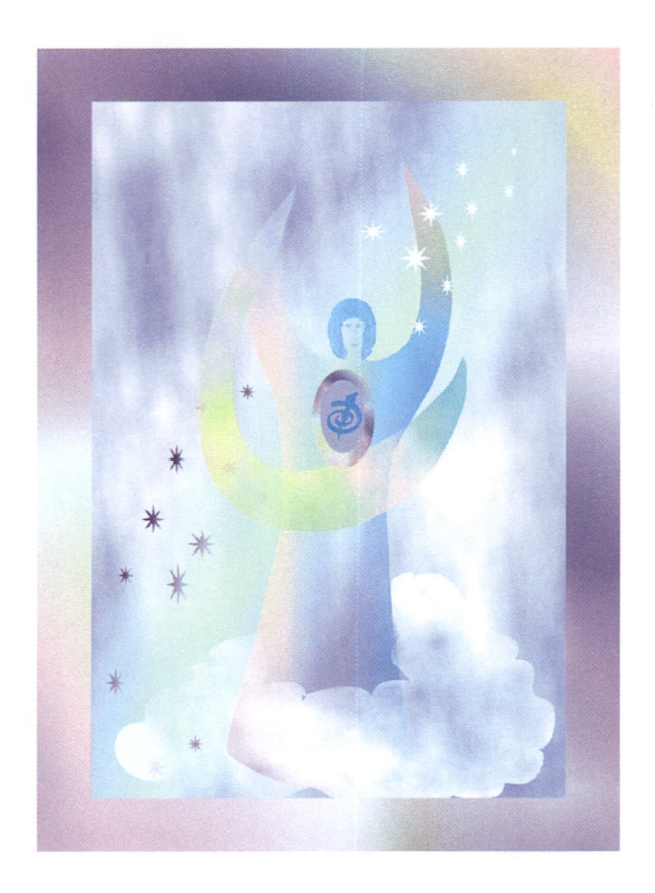

16.Ripples is an art image for the person who is able to send out ripples across the pond to touch the lives of so many. A small step along the road for one soul can also help so many others we have known and loved in past times. As the ripples from our steps begin to spread across the pond their effects are felt by so many across the world and the whole world becomes lighter.

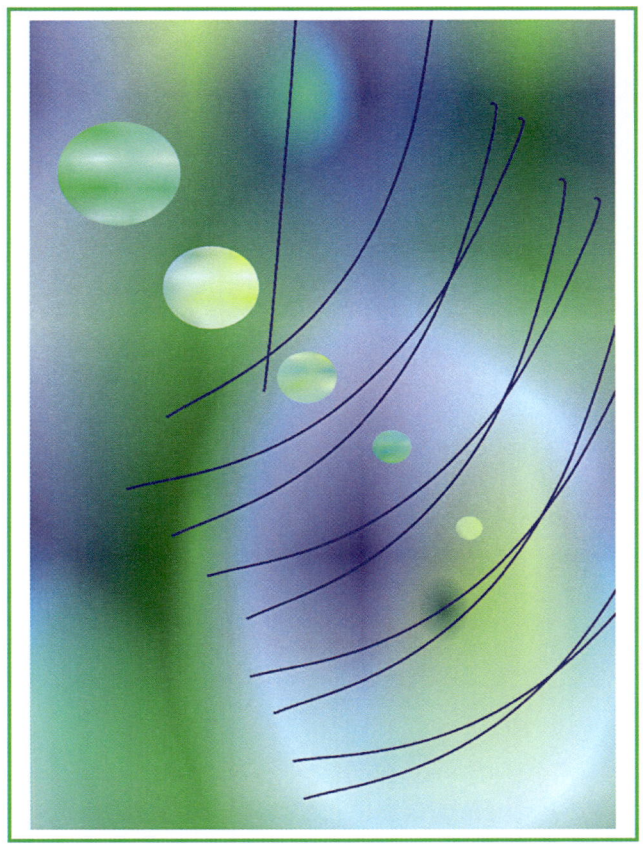

17. Samuse is one of the Angels of the Rainbow where the pot of gold is to be found.   This person may imagine being under attack at any number of different levels. This creates fear in the soul. With Samuse in life the imaginary barbs soften into balls of cotton wool which fall gently to the earth.

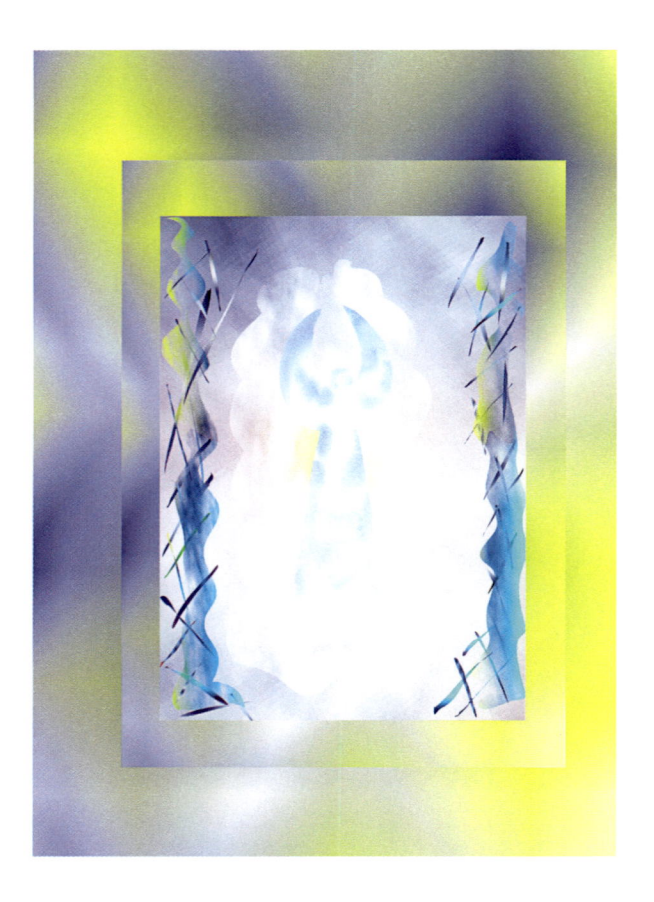

18. Serenity is an enchantment image for the person who has felt the need to erect barriers to keep others out. With these angels around the man made barriers begin to soften. The stones that were previously erected can change into beautiful flowers of peace and serenity.

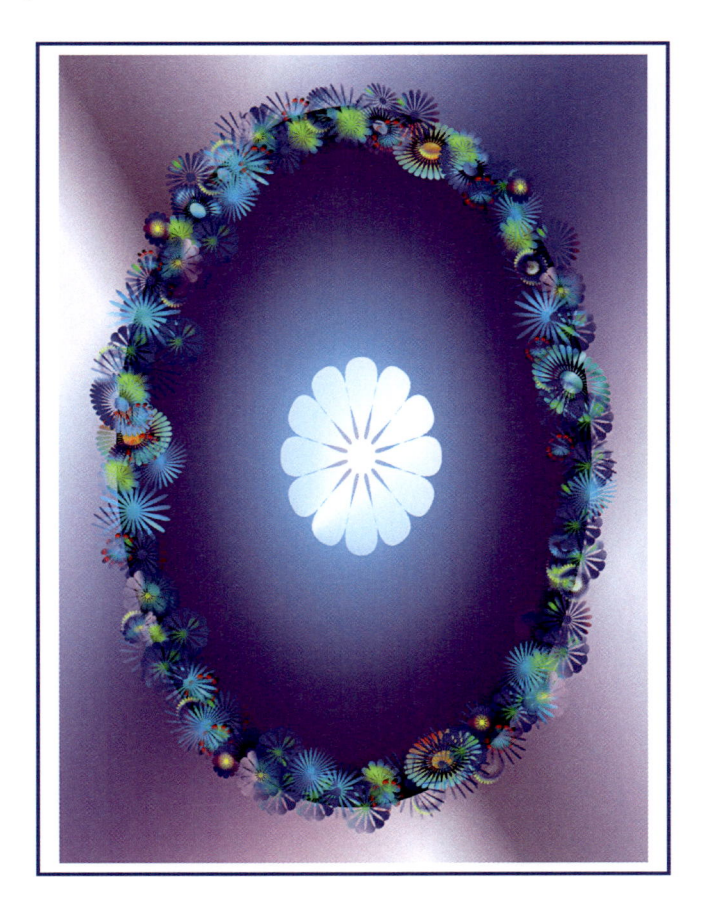

If we keep these fears inside then they can begin to upset the delicate balance of many organs.

19. Spiked is a moonlight dream image for the person who feels as if something intangible is holding them down. This is usually their imagination based on fears from early days or early nightmares which still have a power to affect the soul. The responses within the child were based on fears from parents or the church rather than fears based on reality.

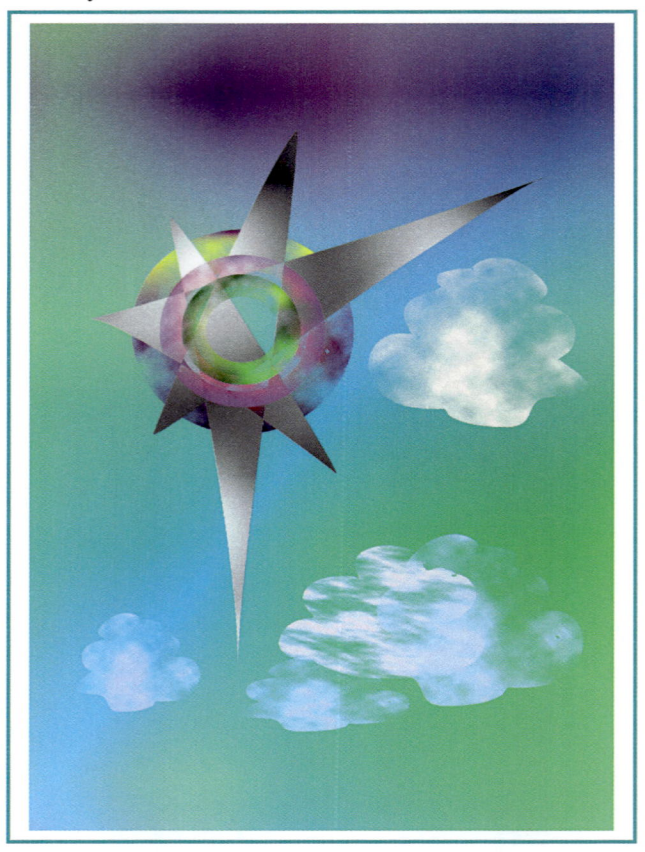

Imagine the spikes slowly loosening and becoming shorter and softer with less power to cause damage.

20. Tzeoreth is the Angel of the Imagination for the soul born between Jan 14th and Jan 17th. He is the angel for obstacles and facing our innermost 'demons'. For this soul the biggest demon is often the fear of the spirits themselves. Tzeoreth lessens this fear and allows the 'demons' to see the light of day. There is no fear greater than fear itself.

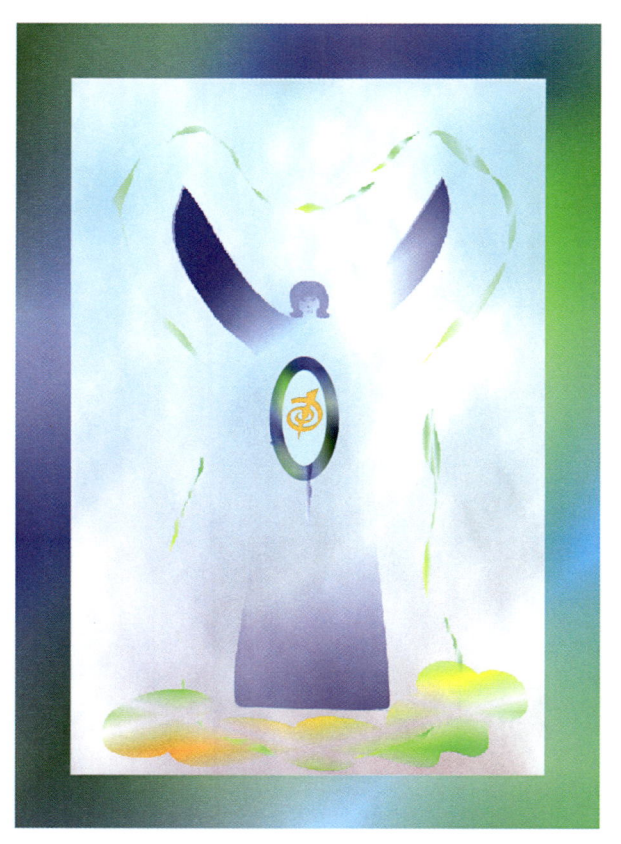

21. Unity is one of the Angels of the Matrix and from the early days on the planet. She is the angel for the god inside us all. This god like all gods is immortal and survives from one life to the next. There is no end just a gentle cycle, where we remeet old friends and lovers again and again, until we have learnt all life's lessons.

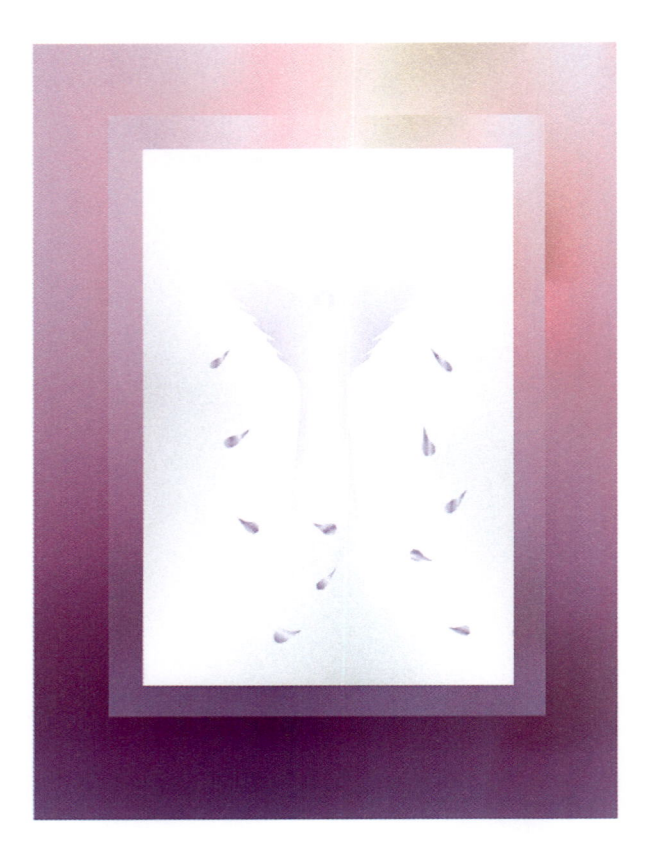

22. Verena is one of the Angels of Innocence and of childhood days when life seemed easier and the world new and exciting. These are the angels of sharing with friends and the sheer enjoyment of the simple things in life. Verena is experimenting with the patterns she can make with her feathers and is totally absorbed in the moment.

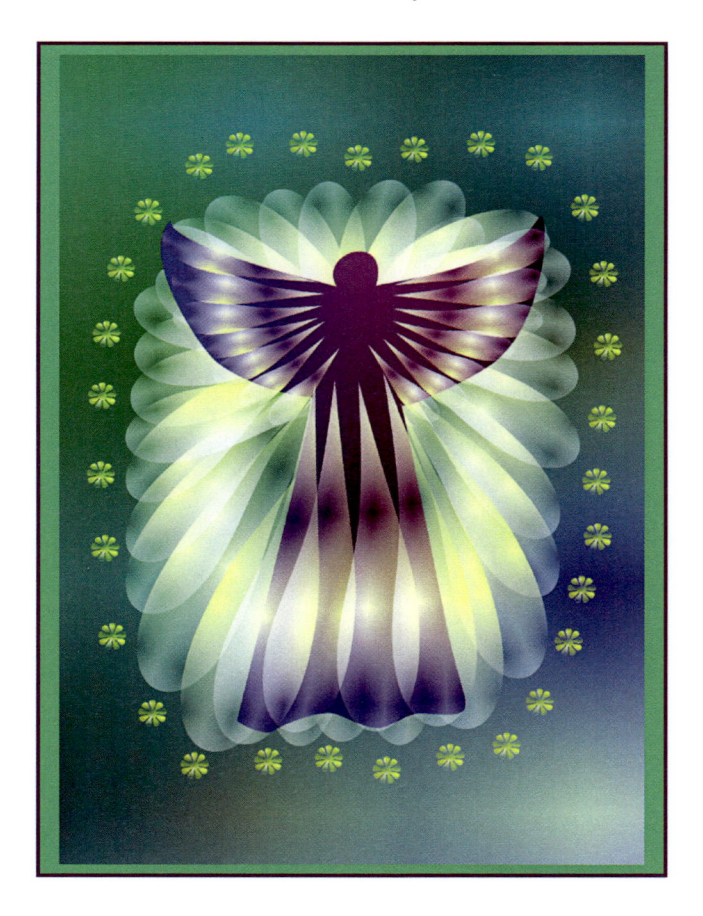

23. Vineas is one of the Alchemy Angels who have the power to transmute our thoughts into nuggets of gold.

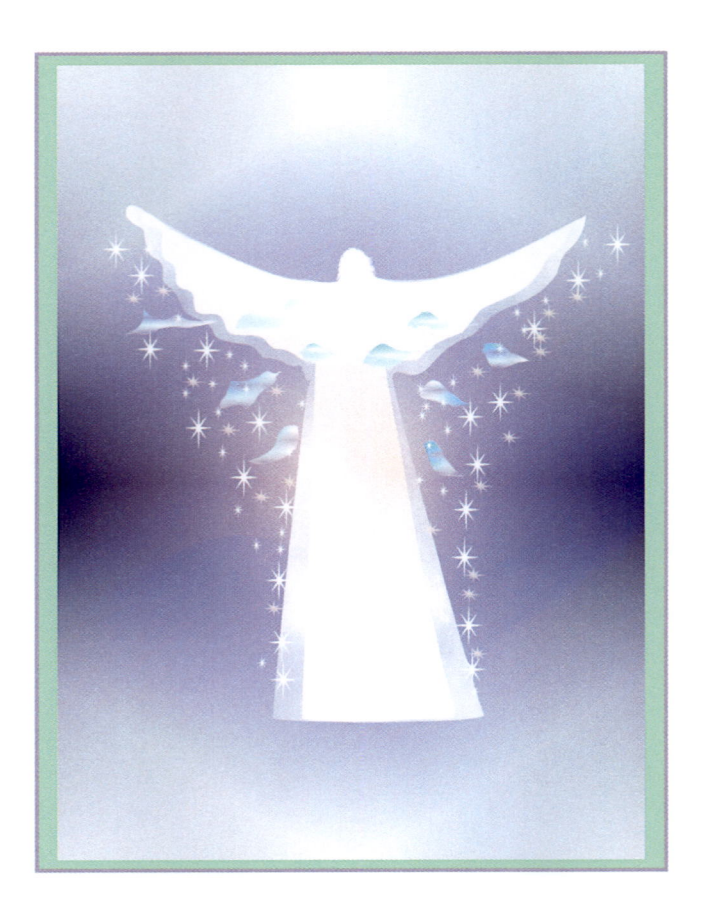

Her message is

'don't settle for the mundane when glory is within your grasp'

Images of Excitement

21. This person appears to need order an stability in their life. If you can allow the boxes to topple over they can break and set you free.

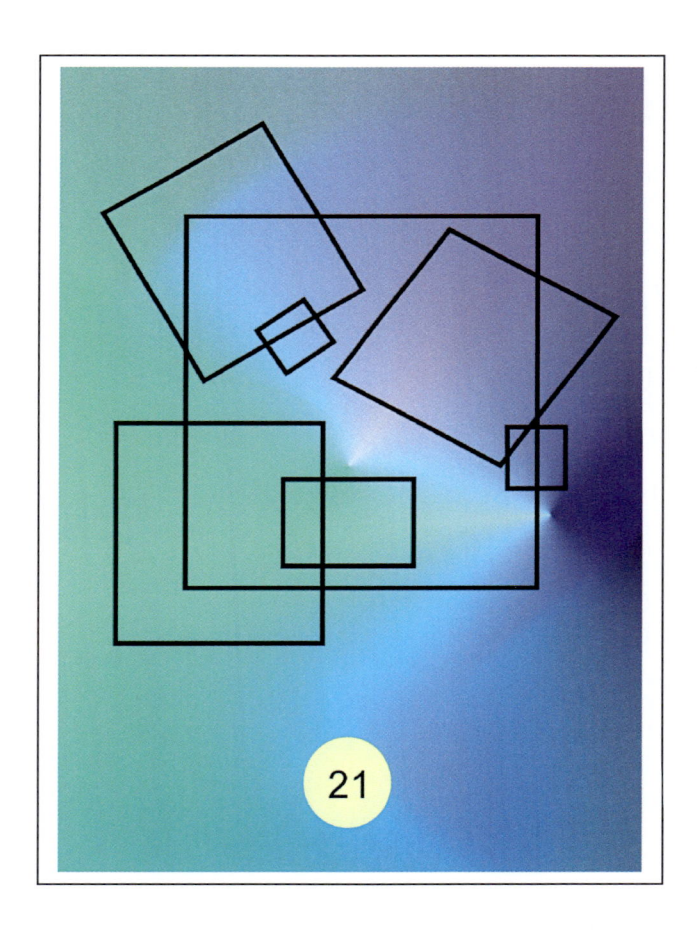

52. This person dreams of freedom but their sense of responsibility holds them back so they continue to dream in the nights but cannot turn this into reality.

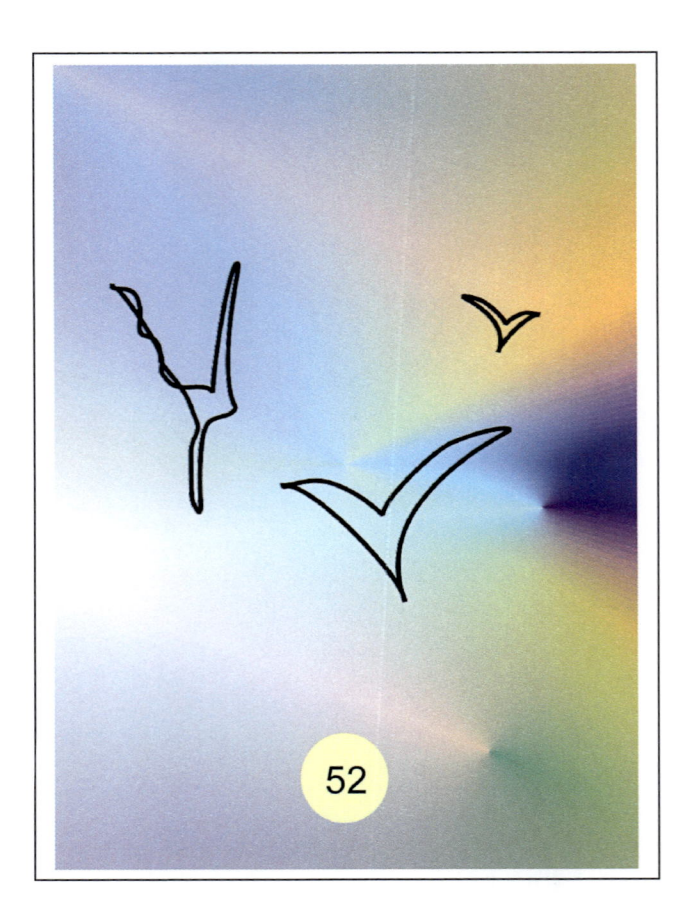

73. These are the inner tears which are never shed but remain inside affecting the water balance of the body.

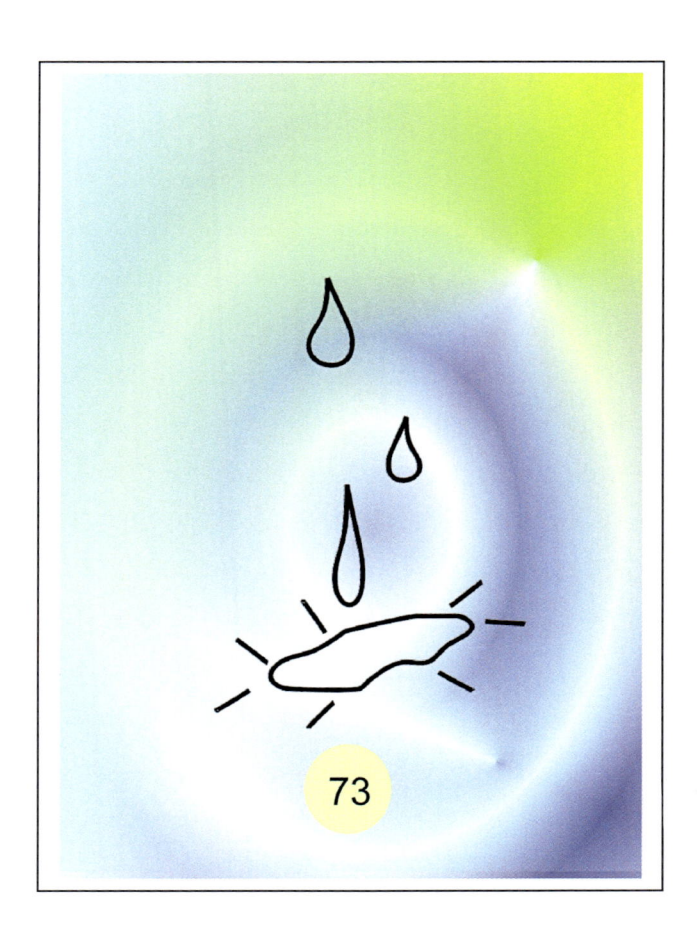

13. The Future

Our responses to events in life define us and allow others to see the truth in who we are. We can all wallow in the energies of our birth time and fail to follow the guidance from above and turn away from our destiny or we can allow these angels and art images to guide us from our own exile in the wilderness. When we invite these angels of the Zodiac into our lives then we are prepared to change and make great strides forward. As these angels begin to heal our problems they also begin to alter our perceptions of reality. This is a part of the Universal Harmonic Healing as the universe helps us to restore the energy body to the state it was in at the start of time long before the person ever stood on the solid ground of the Earth. Harmonic refers to the gentle harmonising of emotions as they flow through the body and in the process they are healed by the angels and returned to us in a brilliant incandescent state.

Patterns have long existed as we live out countless lives and they may make us feel safe for we have survived this pattern and can do so again. Life is not about repeating mistakes it is about learning and making changes for the future incredible. The Capricorn person is born feeling incredibly responsible for others and feels pushed along their pathway. This person wants to find their long term dreams or destiny and walk this path to the very end. Like so many people today they may allow their ideas to be squashed by well meaning people but in so doing they have suppressed the core of the Capricorn person and dowsed their internal passions. Whenever this drive to succeed is hidden away then the body begins to respond to the cold as it continues to want clarity but is unable to find amazing solutions to problems.

The Capricorn person may be thought of as the natural clairsentient, leader and inventor of the world as they always feel responsible for the actions of others. For every person it is important to find one's passion again for through this great joy can be found and a sense of belonging and or altruistically helping others. The human is always master of their own destiny and holds the keys to the kingdom high above the world. This does not mean that in every life the person has to make a majestic sacrifice or achieve tremendous goals but in one life every person will find a way to follow their dreams to glory. If this life is not for you just relax and enjoy the ride into the sunset and have fun for the rest of your days with friends and loved ones.

Summary Sheet for The Capricorn Individual

The energies for this individual are based on the cold and the energies of the mid winter
These energies are also those of the kidney channel from Traditional Chinese medicine, in particular the energy flows around the channel as it flows through the brain.
Ayurvedic vata, apaana, udana
Chakra—throat
Organs affected are the kidneys, the ureters and the muscles of the channel
Colours are various shades of blue
Challenge in this life is to regain the courage to do what is necessary and to find a deep inner faith which will never let the person down
The receptor cells – smooth muscles in the skin and smooth muscle of genitourinary tract, osmoreceptors in hypothalamus, receptors for renin, aldosterone and ANP
Bach Remedy 1- mimulus
2- larch
3- gentian
Tissue salts to help are silica
Homeopathic – arnica, belladonna and silica
Crystal blue lace agate, angelite, moonstone, blue fluorite, blue topaz. Chalcedony, celestine
Time of maximum energy 5 – 7 am
Time of lowered energy 5 – 7 pm